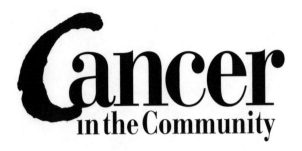

Cancer
in the Community

Smithsonian Series in Ethnographic Inquiry

Ivan Karp and William Merrill, Series Editors

Ethnography as fieldwork, analysis, and literary form is the distinguishing feature of modern anthropology. Guided by the assumption that anthropological theory and ethnography are inextricably linked, this series is devoted to exploring the ethnographic enterprise.

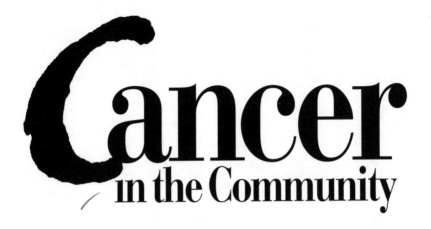

Cancer
in the Community

Class and Medical Authority

Martha Balshem

Smithsonian Institution Press
Washington and London

Copy Editor: Joanne S. Ainsworth
Production Editor: Duke Johns
Designer: Janice Wheeler

Library of Congress Cataloging-in-Publication Data
Balshem, Martha Levittan.
  Cancer in the community : class and medical authority /
Martha Balshem.
  p.   cm.
Includes bibliographical references and index.
ISBN 1–56098–250–0 (cloth : alk. paper).—ISBN 1-
56098–251–9 (paper : alk. paper)
  1. Cancer—Prevention—Social aspects.   2. Health
education—Pennsylvania—Philadelphia.   3. Health education—
Social aspects.   4. Health education—Political aspects.   5.
Social medicine.   6. Cancer—Pennsylvania—Philadelphia.   I.
Title.
  [DNLM: 1. Health Education. 2. Knowledge, Attitudes,
Practice. 3. Neoplasms—psychology. 4. Social Perception.
QZ 200 B196t]
  RA645.C3B35   1993
306.4′61′08623—dc20
DNLM/DLC
for Library of Congress   92–48963

British Library Cataloguing-in-Publication Data is available

Manufactured in the United States of America
00 99 98 97 96 95 94 93   5 4 3 2 1

⊗The paper used in this publication meets the minimum
requirements of the American National Standard for Permanence of
Paper for Printed Library Materials Z39.48–1984.

To James Dolan

CONTENTS

Preface   **ix**

Acknowledgments   **xv**

1. **Defining the Topic   1**

2. **The Study Community   13**

3. **Project CAN-DO   55**

4. **A Cancer Death   91**

5. **Meaning for the Anthropologist   125**

6. **Changing the Victim   141**

Notes   **149**

References   **157**

Index   **170**

PREFACE

This book is about negotiating professional authority. The professional authority with which I begin my discussion is that of scientific medicine. Critiques of the medical profession come easily. In the social science literature, medicine has served as the model for critiques of professional authority in general. In this book, too, discussion of the authority of medicine predominates. My purpose, however, is a broader discussion of the roots of professional authority in general and of what both professionals and lay people learn through the experience of such authority.

Medical authority, my beginning point, is a complex phenomenon. It is well understood, and can be seen in the stories I tell in this book, that expressions of medical authority are often loaded with meanings about other things—truth and legitimacy, power and resistance, self and identity. Thus, an examination of medical authority leads naturally to wider topics. My own wider topic here concerns the images of superiority and inferiority that inform all professional practice.

At different points in the book, I speak directly to different professional audiences. Health educators are most directly addressed in Chapter 3; physicians in Chapter 4; and anthropologists in Chapter 5. I hope, however, that all readers—especially my colleagues in anthropology—

will feel addressed by my entire effort and that I will also find an audience among others who have felt or thought about the authority of medicine, or any professional authority, as a burden.

My medical focus is on the disease we call cancer. The word *cancer* is actually a rubric for more than one hundred different diseases. Nevertheless, in this book, I will speak as if cancer were one discrete entity, because that is how the word is used in lay discourse, and the usage dominates debate between scientists and the public.

In the chapters to follow, I will describe conflicts within and between professional and lay systems of belief about cancer. I will describe how these conflicts are expressed by and about residents of Tannerstown (a pseudonym), a high-cancer-risk, European-American working-class neighborhood in Philadelphia. The conflicts I will describe involve the powerful authoritative stance of professional scientific medicine; the powerful cultural resistance posed by Tannerstown residents; and the uneasily derivative and internally conflicted professional positions of both health educators and applied anthropologists.

This account is based on my three and one-half years of work at the Fox Chase Cancer Center in Philadelphia. For my first two years at Fox Chase, I worked in Tannerstown and nearby neighborhoods as a health educator for a cancer education project called Project CAN-DO. This constricted my view of neighborhood life. Although we described Project CAN-DO as a general health promotion program, it was widely understood that we were focused primarily on cancer prevention. Partly because Fox Chase Cancer Center is not well known in Tannerstown, many people we met were not quite sure where we were from. We were identified variously as being from Fox Chase Cancer Center, from a well-regarded community hospital in the Fox Chase area, from the American Cancer Society, or from the vaguely identified entity "the cancer research." Nonetheless, it was clear in the minds of Tannerstowners that we were focused on advising people to change their lifestyles to reduce their cancer risk. This colored my relationships with people.

Furthermore, my workload as a health educator was heavy and dictated how I spent most of my time in the neighborhood. For two years, I gave talks to elementary and junior high school students in public and Catholic schools. I got to know schoolteachers and principals, ate in teachers' lunchrooms, and attended Home and School (parent-teacher association) meetings. I worked with Project CAN-DO advisory board members, gave presentations at senior citizens' clubs, conducted and attended focus groups on various health topics, and worked with community activists to organize special programs. Along the way, I made friends. But my informal time in the community was always limited. In the following year and a half, my administrative duties at Fox Chase increased and I was in the community less.

During none of this time did I define myself as an anthropologist "in the field." My formal data are therefore thinner than my experience. In particular, I have few field notes on which to depend. Therefore, in my representation of community voices, I have depended heavily on transcripts of twenty-five formal interviews of neighborhood women, and eight focus groups, done at various times, some of which involved male participants. In the narrative of this book I present quotations, sometimes lengthy, from these transcripts. I have used this material judiciously, with care that quoted material should represent themes that my experiences and observations taught me were important.

Throughout, I have changed or omitted specific details that might have led to the identification of individual respondents. In most cases, I have used pseudonyms for people, places, and institutions.

My relationship with Tannerstown was special; my view of Tannerstown is correspondingly partial. My focus is on the politicalization of cancer and the ways in which talking about cancer translates into talk about other things. This, my experience richly documents.

In Chapter 1, I describe ravelings and unravelings that shaped my various analyses and brought me to my bottom-line questions about the ethics of professional authority. In Chapter 2, I briefly trace the history of industry in Tannerstown and look at how debate about cancer and pollution has been woven into images of Tannerstown held by various groups of people. In Chapter 3, I detail local interpretations of Project CAN-DO and the meanings of the local critique of scientific authority. This critique focuses on the power to define truth and on the arrogance of those who would devalue community lifeways and worldviews. The focus of Chapter 4 is a medical case history in which the same critique is played out in the clinic, in the context of the cancer death of a Tannerstown resident. In this case, realities of life and death transform the emotional tone of the debate. In Chapter 5, I look at my own role as an anthropologist and at the threads of professional authority and self-identity with which I weave my images of the community and of the professions of health education, medicine, and anthropology. In Chapter 6, I discuss the roots of professional authority and attempt an answer to the emotional and ethical dilemma that assuming such authority can create.

Throughout, I set my analysis aggressively into the framework of my own felt experience. In doing so, I have documented the way in which my analysis has developed—pushed forward at every turn by my efforts to be emotionally honest with myself. This is, as many readers will appreciate, a difficult task. I hope I have succeeded and that the book will stand as an argument for the usefulness of reflexivity.

Another issue requires discussion in this Preface, and that is the relationship of my work to the literature in health promotion and health education. As readers in those fields will be aware, the critique of health education that I present in this book is not original. Many important scholars in health education have voiced the same critique that I have concerning the concept of individual responsibility for health, presented incisive arguments against victim blaming in health education practice, and moved from philosophical questions to programmatic ones.[1] To the literature in health education, I have aimed to contribute not a new concern but an ethnographic case study of the challenges involved in making changes that many in health education define as necessary.

During the time that I have been writing about cancer, many colleagues in health education (and some outside that field) have raised two major objections to me about my work. I will address both of these objections here and hope that they are also addressed throughout the book.

The first objection I commonly hear is that the beliefs about cancer that I describe are not unique to Tannerstown. This is very true. As I discuss later, these beliefs are common in many societies and have existed in the United States at least as far back as the 1800s. I do not claim that these beliefs are unique to Tannerstown, or to working-class communities in general. Still, in Tannerstown—a working-class neighborhood with a high cancer rate—cancer has become a strongly politicized issue. The cancer beliefs that residents express are not unique, but they are elaborated and expressed with insight and emotion that are particularly vivid. In my view, this is partly animated by the distrust of authority that is particularly strong in many working-class environments. But I do not trace the existence of the beliefs themselves to these same environments.

The second objection that is commonly made to my work on cancer is that I do not suggest concrete take-home messages for cancer-control practice. My work is very critical of health education in general, in the sense that I see basic structural conflicts besetting the field and impeding its progress. But, then, what is my bottom line? As one critic put it, do I mean to say that health education has no place in the effort to reduce the burden of cancer in this country? This question is vexing, because I have no concrete suggestions to offer. I believe that quantum leaps in the effectiveness of cancer-control programs could be achieved if the social and cultural contexts of professional practice were changed. The same is true for clinical medicine. Many health educators and physicians know this, and with greater analytical and emotional force than I do. I know it most clearly about anthropology, my own field, for which I still have few concrete suggestions for reform. I only hope that my book will help to fill in various roadmaps by providing a concrete picture of the personal and cultural complexities that changing professions will entail.

ACKNOWLEDGMENTS

I am deeply grateful to the people of Tannerstown (a pseudonym), and other neighborhoods in the river wards area of Philadelphia, for the welcome they gave me, both as a health educator and as an anthropologist. I hope that they will find my portrayal of them in this book to be accurate and that they will be glad to read what I have written.

I owe an enormous debt of gratitude to the woman I refer to as Jennifer, whose narrative about her husband's death forms a significant part of Chapter 4. It was in the process of writing her story, and constructing my own commentary on her insights, that I began to think about writing this book. I am sure that some of her work with me was emotionally difficult for her, and I have been inspired by her determination to speak out for the benefit of others. I hope that she will be pleased with the result of our work together.

I am also extremely grateful to the physician I refer to in Chapter 4 and thereafter as Dr. Hughes and to his colleagues and staff at the institution I refer to as Hospital F. Dr. Hughes gave me a truly collegial welcome and generously spoke of his medical practice in emotionally open terms.

Ivan Karp encouraged me early on to conceive of this material as a book. He has encouraged me throughout with just the right advice for the struggling writer. As always, he has been a great source of insight regarding conceptual matters and has understood exactly where I needed to rewrite and expand what I was saying. Each contact with him has pushed me to do better work.

Zili Amsel, Mary B. Daly, and Paul F. Engstrom read an early draft of the manuscript and were generous with their insights. I have attempted to do their comments justice, and the book has benefited through this process. I thank them for their considerable time and effort.

Throughout my work on cancer education, I have had the support of many remarkable people. Emily Martin gave me generous assistance when I was trying, years ago, to draw together a line of research regarding this topic. Her own work has inspired me, as it has many others. Zili Amsel, formerly of Project CAN-DO, hired me at Fox Chase Cancer Center, supported my efforts to do ethnographic work, and showed faith in me through many turns. Barbara Rimer helped me to appreciate the central ethical devotion to the public health that inspires the best in health education research and was an honest and generous guide in difficult times. Paul F. Engstrom gave me an opportunity that changed my professional life and then gave me the support I needed to swim rather than sink. I have been fortunate to have had the support of such people.

I am grateful to Mary B. Daly, M.D.; Michael H. Levy, M.D.; Joan James, Physician Assistant–Certified; and, again, to Paul F. Engstrom, M.D., for allowing me to observe clinical and hospital practice in medical oncology. This experience, although limited by my own time constraints, helped to orient me to issues in medical oncology. I am particularly grateful to Mary B. Daly for pointing me toward issues for further research.

Stephen Workman, my dear comrade in the field, has shared many of my triumphs and woes. I hope I have learned something from his sense of perspective. Michael Herzfeld, ever generous with his time and insight, pointed me in the right direction at a critical time. Paul L. Jamison, as always, has been my academic home base, and a source of great encouragement. For friendship, good advice, and intellectual companionship, I am also indebted to Jane K. Cowan, Katherine A.

Dettwyler, Robert Leopold, Caryn Lerman, Ronald Myers, C. Tracy Orleans, Elliott Shore, and Beverly Sibthorpe. Thomas Biolsi merits special mention for endless discussions about forms of domination, for introducing me to Caffe Nikko, and for many other acts of true collegiality. I would also like to thank Helen Anderson, Doris Gillespie, Thomas J. Mason, Leslie McBride, Gary Oxman, Bradley P. Stoner, and Bruce Trock for assistance with background research; and Colleen Burke and Linda Fleisher for their friendship and support. I reserve a special thanks for Andrew Balshem, more than a friend and coworker, with whom I have been fortunate to have had two distinct but equally wonderful relationships.

I am pleased to thank Constance J. Cash and Joanne Murray for expert administrative assistance, and for transcription of the highest quality. I am also pleased to thank Leanne Pinniger and Margaret Meibohm, both excellent research assistants, and Jennifer Scarboro, who conducted a valuable literature search. In addition, I would like to thank Patricia Potrzebowski and Cynthia Morgan of the Pennsylvania Division of Health Statistics and Research and David Segal of the Philadelphia City Planning Commission for their generous assistance in providing statistical data regarding the Philadelphia community; the *Guide* newspaper, published in Philadelphia, Pennsylvania, for permission to quote from the column "by Dan" and to reprint one column almost in its entirety; and *Philadelphia Magazine,* also published in Philadelphia, Pennsylvania, for granting me permission to quote extensively from that publication.

I am very grateful to Daniel Goodwin of the Smithsonian Institution Press for all his help, for his unflagging enthusiasm about this book, and for his kindly patience throughout the publication process. I would also like to thank Joanne S. Ainsworth for editing the manuscript with such loving care.

Some of the material in this book has been presented previously. Much of Chapter 3 appeared in article form in the *American Ethnologist* (Balshem 1991a); this material benefited greatly from suggestions by Donald Brenneis, Kristin Fossum, and four anonymous reviewers. My analysis has also benefited from discussions following presentations to the Department of Anthropology, Oregon State University;

the American Studies Seminar, Portland State University; the Department of Health Education and Health Promotion, Kaiser-Permanente, Portland, Oregon; and the Anthropology Students Association at Portland State University. Classroom discussions and other communications with Portland State University students have been a continuing source of energy and fresh insight.

Some of the original research on which this book is based was supported by Public Health Service Grant no. CA34856 and was conducted while I was employed by Fox Chase Cancer Center, Philadelphia. Further research was supported by grants from the Faculty Development Committee and the Research and Publications Committee, both of Portland State University. I am grateful for the support of all agencies. I am also grateful to Michael Reardon, Provost of Portland State University, a creative facilitator of faculty research.

Through the years, discussions with Howard Balshem, my favorite Philadelphia native, have helped me to focus my thinking, keep my perspective, and maintain my self-confidence. I hope that I can support his academic endeavors as well as he has supported mine. My daughter, Rebecca, five years old, has helped by being so excited about "mommy's book." My son, Steven, two years old, has helped by giving me his unconditional love. My family has allowed me the joy of writing this book and has endured my many absences with little open complaint.

I will reserve my final thanks for my mother, who can take pride in my accomplishments as her own, and for my father, who gave me enough love to last past a lifetime.

DEFINING THE TOPIC 1

*[T]here is no such thing as a merely given, or simply available, starting
point: beginnings have to be made for each project in such a way as to
enable what follows from them.*
Edward W. Said, *Orientalism*

I am on the same level as they are. Or better.
Tannerstown resident

At the 1986 meeting of the American Anthropological Association
(AAA), I presented a paper as part of a session on medical discourse. I
was ninth on a panel of ten. The papers were uniformly interesting,
and the large audience stayed for the whole session. My later recon-
struction reflects my own strong emotional experience of the session.
What stands out in my imagination is this: early in the session, a paper
was presented on the ethnoanatomy of a people in Zaire (Kornfield
1986). The presenter passed out a sketch to the audience, detailing
how some people in Zaire believe that the child in utero is connected
to the outside world through a tube to the mother's navel. The author
related this, along with other elements of ethnoanatomy, to indigenous explanations of the physical complaints of pregnant women. The
argument was detailed and interesting, and the audience followed the
diagram and analysis seriously and intently. Other interesting papers
followed. Then it was my turn. I described the cancer beliefs of some
residents of Tannerstown, a European-American working-class neighborhood in Philadelphia (Balshem et al. 1986). I reported to the audience that many residents of this community believe that a bump or a
bruise on the breast can cause cancer, that surgery can cause cancer to
spread, that there is cancer inside everybody, and that it is partly fate

that dictates who develops the disease. Much to my astonishment, the audience reacted by laughing, not at any intended witticisms of my own, but at the beliefs of the people I was describing. Feeling a little disoriented, I pushed through to the end of the presentation and was applauded loudly—for, it seemed, the unanticipated amusement value of my presentation. Afterward, several people approached me and told me that the people *they* worked with held precisely the same beliefs. These colleagues appeared to find it amazing and somehow wonderful to have these things described in a paper at the AAA. All in all, the experience was unsettling.

When I returned to my home institution—at that time, Fox Chase Cancer Center in Philadelphia—I described to my colleagues in the Division of Cancer Control the audience's reaction to my paper. I discovered that my experience was not unique and that presentations to health psychologists and oncologists had engendered similar hilarity. Through this, I came to suspect that the meaning of the incident at the AAA meeting was related not only to the culture of anthropology but also to some element of the general relationship between professionals and working-class people.

For years I kept this incident on the edge of my consciousness. I had many disquieting questions. Had my audience been caught unawares by a description of nonscientific beliefs within our own society? Were some anthropologists from the United States nervous about studies done too close to home? But surely, we have a long tradition of such studies. Did my audience interpret the European-American urban working class as Self or Other? Could we extend our central professional value of respect for cultural differences to groups within our own society? I thought about these things through the next few years while I worked at Fox Chase and had limited contact with colleagues in anthropology. But I never really felt that I understood what had happened. Something was missing in my perception.

During the next few years I was very busy at Fox Chase. My experiences there were similar to those that many anthropologists have faced in the "applied world." I was one of a group of eight investigators, all with doctoral degrees—two specialists in health education, two health psychologists, two epidemiologists, one sociologist, and myself, the one anthropologist. The group was constituted, if not quite officially then certainly in practice, as the Department of Behavioral Science. Behavioral science paradigms informed our work, and ethnographic method was not always well understood. The researchers were for the most part talented, dedicated people, motivated by a sense that their work was important and worthwhile. I did not need to hear very many horror stories from people in the Tannerstown community—stories about women who had hidden their breast lump from everyone for years, for instance—before I began to construct the view that resistance to the recommendations of scientific cancer control was a tragedy. My colleagues at Fox Chase clearly saw their purpose as the prevention of suffering—specifically, lowering cancer morbidity and mortality—through educating people to change their lifestyles. Our central messages were: quit smoking, improve your diet, and schedule cancer-screening tests at recommended intervals.

Who could be against that? I was not against it. And yet, as my professional identity at Fox Chase developed, I began to experience a growing sense of dis-ease. This was engendered at least in part by negative feelings I encountered from among the residents of Tannerstown.

Tannerstown is, as mentioned above, a European-American working-class community. Fox Chase had started educational programs there because cancer rates in Tannerstown are very high. As I will describe later, Tannerstowners resisted the message that these high cancer rates were associated with their personal habits. They pointed a finger instead at air pollution from the large chemical plants next to the community and at occupational exposure, air pollution from heavy street traffic, and chemical adulteration of food and water. As representatives of the cancer center, we sought to deflect this concern and stressed lifestyle changes to reduce cancer risk. Privately, we acknowledged our own feelings or suspicions that the profound pollution we observed in the community was somehow linked to the high cancer rates. We said to each other that this did not present us with a moral dilemma, because in any case, people were well advised to quit smoking, improve their diets, and get regular cancer tests. The risks associated with smoking and diet might well act synergistically with risks from pollution, and finding cancer early is critical regardless of how the cancer first developed. But I and some of my confidants at the cancer center turned the question over and over in our minds. Was it valid to tell people to change their lifestyles? Was the behavioral science enterprise manipulative? Or was this issue unimportant compared with the prospect of preventing, through our work, even one case of cancer, or one cancer death?

CONFLICT: AN INITIAL FRAMEWORK

My sense of ambivalence about my professional role was profound, and the questions I asked myself felt unresolvable. Perhaps partly because the issues were so painful, I did not pursue them as a central topic while I was at Fox Chase. Instead, I worked at constructing conceptual frameworks through which to view not myself but the community and professional worlds around me.[1]

The central research goal of the Fox Chase cancer-control group was to develop strategies to encourage changes in individual behavior, to lower individual risk of cancer. With much uneasiness, I accepted that as my central research problem. I sought the approval of my colleagues. I wanted to show that anthropology could contribute importantly to our understanding of health beliefs and behaviors. But my internal, more personal framework was critical of the health-education stance. In my private view of the conflict between health educators and community residents, I saw the views of both parties as problematic. The conflict between these two views may be elucidated by looking at the general representations that many medical professionals and working-class lay people construct of each other.

Professional Representations of the Working Class

On one side of the conflict are professional representations of the working class. For many professional observers of industrial society, the working class is the Other within. Even the phrasing "the working class" indicates a monolith, a piece of structure, an institution about which one can generalize. Seemingly objective generalizations about the working class are often loaded with assumptions. In the United States, class status is generally measured through some combination of occupation, education, and income. All three measures are riddled with problems of definition and have an inexact and variable relation to each other and to other measures of class status. These measures point most clearly to a stereotype: a low-income blue-collar worker with a modest formal education.

This stereotype supports higher-order assumptions about the working class. One of the most central of these is that working-class people are failures. In the United States, where we are regarded as captains of our own fate, relative poverty is seen as an individual defect. Charles Valentine (1968) and William Ryan (1976) wrote many years ago that lay people and professionals in the United States tend to "blame the victim" by locating the reason for poverty in the characteristics of the poor. This critique is still relevant.

Even those who would stand as advocates of the working class are influenced by the tendency to blame the victim. With industrial decline, the working class is seen less often as a powerful potential for transformation and more often as a social ill to be cured. Western intellectuals agonize over this. Some write with despair of brooding poverty that devastates the working-class spirit; others celebrate working-class expressive culture as a powerful font of resistance.[2] Theoretical debates rage. Does the working class resist? Or are they defeated right through to the soul? Such debate is animated by the angst of the intellectual whose faith in the working class ex machina is shaken.

For many public-policy planners, the working class can be written even more crudely as a problem. Social planners speak of the "persistence of poverty"—a phrase that communicates the premise that the poor are an adversary to the best efforts of the planners. The problem is identified as being located within working-class people themselves. Too often, social workers, politicians, and educators see working-class status as a problem that needs correction.

These views find expression within the culture of medicine. It is a central tenet of modern preventive medicine that people bear responsibility for their sickness, through control over their lifestyles. In any case of sickness, the patient's life may be judged, and there is a feeling of morality in this judgment. Did the patient cause the disease? Was the patient's lifestyle at fault? In the field of cancer control, enthusiasm for the promotion of lifestyle change is animated by widely respected estimates that 60–85 percent of all cancers are attributable to lifestyle factors (Doll and Peto 1981:1205; Greenwald and Sondik 1986:15).

With regard to lifestyle and health, working-class people in particular are often judged as lacking.[3] To professional health educators, the working class is the final frontier: they still smoke, take drugs, eat high-fat diets, drink too much alcohol, and fail to go for regular checkups. Much of the literature on health promotion implies that good health for the working class demands the elimination of traditional lifestyles and beliefs, and adherence to the recommendations of scientific experts in health promotion. In the clinic, too, working-class people are cast negatively. Negative judgments underlie common analytical concepts used in community and clinical health research, such as "working-class fatalism," "the troublesome patient," and "the angry patient," and animate the vast literature on the problem of noncompliance.[4]

Working-Class Representations of the Medical Profession

On the other side of the conflict, I saw lay views of the medical profession. These, too, tend toward gross generalities: physicians are arrogant, controlling, and care only about making a lot of money. Most of us are familiar with these popular stereotypes. Very often, people do not see their *own* physicians in this way but still see the medical profession as a whole in this light.

An important element in this negative view of the medical profession is that physicians and their allies are seen as having excessive power to control knowledge. In the lay image, medical professionals control the research decisions that determine what comes to be known, decree that only their own knowledge is legitimate, and jealously withhold that knowledge from patients and from lay people in general. For many lay people, contact with the medical-care system has at some point involved the felt experience of a loss of personal authority. These experiences are often dramatic and terrifying, because our bodies and sometimes even our lives are involved.

Academic critiques of the medical profession are a special case of these lay representations and focus on the same themes. Medical social scientists have described in elaborate detail the physician's power to confer or deny legitimacy to particular interpretations of patient sign, symptom, and behavior; charged that through the distinction between scientific and folk knowledge, lay interpretations are cast as illegitimate and inconvenient counterpoints to real medical knowledge; documented that the dialogue through which physicians decide whose knowledge is real is kept secret from patients; shown that questions initiated by the patient are often not answered or are not answered readily or sufficiently; and indicated that physicians resent and discourage patient self-diagnosis and keep tight control over the flow of information onto the patient's chart (for instance, Cicourel 1983; Greene et al. 1986; Jordan 1977; Steward and Sullivan 1982; West 1983). Such research is often directly inspired by the personal experiences of the researchers.

Working-class people may not see these issues any differently from the way non-working-class people do. In the United States, people of all socioeconomic positions criticize the medical profession for misuse of authority and question the suspect legitimacy of professional claims to knowledge. But working-class people have a vital tradition of criticism, often expressing it in an exceptionally lively manner. This tradition of criticism is an integral theme in working-class culture and is often tied to affirmations of the value of working-class traditions. It is debatable whether these critiques are, when in working-class hands, part of a special font of resistance; but it is true in any case that the working class expresses them with special vigor.

In my working environment at Fox Chase, I saw both sides of the conflict between medical science and the working-class lay public. The cancer-control researchers had designed a number of major programs for working-class populations. This focus was seen as meritorious because in the view of leading cancer-control researchers working-class populations are particularly in need of education and are particularly hard to educate. Tannerstowners offered a strong counterpoint. They did not view themselves as in need of the education being offered and saw the offer itself as evidence of the arrogance of medical science. The conflict was clear, and the framework to which it led drew me to see Tannerstown's critique of medical science as being "right." But affiliating in this way with the community did not ease my sense of discomfort about my work as a health educator. Because medical science could be seen to be arrogant, was it therefore "wrong" to tell people not to smoke? My conflict concerning my own professional role endured.

LIVING CONFLICT

After three years at Fox Chase, I decided to look for a position as an academic anthropologist. The decision was in the main a positive one, based on my decision to develop as an anthropologist and not commit to the role of researcher within the framework of behavioral science. I felt that I would lose something important of myself if I stayed at Fox Chase any longer. I also could not shake my feeling of discomfort with my role at the cancer center—or, maybe more exactly, with living a professional life that I was not understanding clearly. That next year I happily accepted an academic position and began to write about my experiences in cancer control. Over the course of my first academic term, I noted a change in what I was writing. In short, I realized that I had not, in the words of James Scott, been able to "think my way free" (1985:39) to a critical analysis until I had left Fox Chase. As I gained some distance from my conflicts, my gaze turned more toward what my own role at Fox Chase had been.

One day during my second term of teaching, with my first article written and in the mail, I saw a report in *Science News* (Fackelmann 1990) that described the research of Arnis Richters. Richters's research, which involves studies of laboratory animals, suggests that air pollution may reduce the immune system's ability to fight the spread of cancer cells (see discussion in Richters 1988). This implies that in human populations exposed to heavy air pollution, cancer patients may be less likely to survive their disease, leading to higher rates of cancer mortality. It also implies that the immune systems of people who breathe heavily polluted air may be less effective in clearing the bloodstream of the showers of cancer cells that occur after cancer surgery. In other words, surgery might cause cancer to spread. All of this fit the views of cancer causation dominant in Tannerstown. I put the magazine down and felt the bottom drop out of something internally. It was a relief.

I finally realized the extent to which I was still, in a sense, blurring both the community's and my own critique of cancer-control practice. Despite my advocacy of the critique made by community residents— and the strongly critical stance I had taken in my recent article—I was still pushing to the side my own sense of shame and doubt about the role I had assumed in my work in cancer control. At the cancer center, I had entered into a tacit agreement with myself to try on the world view of cancer control, to see how it felt, and to put aside something of myself for the sake of that affiliation. The siren song of medical science was very strong, and I had been willing to adapt and seek acceptance. (Emily Martin reports having similar experiences while doing research on the culture of immunology; see Martin 1989.) For instance, to date, in my written descriptions of community beliefs about cancer, I had felt it necessary to point out that the community critique is *based on* fact—an epistemological category distinctly different from *being* fact. In this and other ways, I had allowed the implication that ultimate knowledge is still always held by medical science. Given this, my advocacy of community views had never really been open and clear and had never successfully put my feelings of professional discomfort to rest. But I had labeled this a personal matter, an emotional matter, and pushed it aside. In doing so, I had pushed aside my thoughts and feelings about one entire side of the conflict I was seeing: the side that was inhabited by health educators and other professionals. As is often done in medical social science, I had rendered the Other (in this case, the working-class community) elaborately and had drawn the professional more thinly, even though that was the role that I myself had lived. My rendering of the discourse between community residents and health educators was, despite my best efforts, still subtly divorced from my own experience. I had constructed my major research interest as the health beliefs of a working-class community and partitioned off my uncomfortable fascination with my own professional life. This was underscored when I began to work on a second article on my cancer-control research, which focused on the medical case history that I present in Chapter 4 of this book. Again, I could represent the conflicts involved from the point of view of the patient's wife (the patient being deceased) but not from the point of view of the physician. In avoiding the physician's emotional experience, I had again avoided the professional's experience of the conflict I was investigating.

I could now revisit the incident of the laughing audience at the AAA meeting. What had been missing from my perception was not related to my analysis of the audience's reaction to me. The questions I was raising about that were good enough. What was missing was an analysis of my reactions to the audience. I had not admitted to myself that I felt uncomfortable about the material I was presenting because I was uncomfortable with my role at the cancer center. When I presented the paper at the AAA meeting, I felt strains in my stance as a health educator and in my stance as an anthropologist. I felt betwixt and between, and honest nowhere. Maybe my audience at the AAA had laughed at a presentation that came uncomfortably close to treating the audience members as subjects of research. But maybe I had also turned aside from studying myself. I had failed to study the professional. I had defined advocacy of the Other—of the working-class community I was working in—as the core of my professional practice. I had defined this advocacy as an appropriate, ethical, and satisfying stance for an anthropologist. I had, in fact, presented an analysis of a conflict to which I myself was a party, without including an analysis of my own role. And it was in an analysis of my own role that the answer to my root questions lay.

Anthropologists, being in the business of representing others, assume a special responsibility to attempt thoughtful self-representation. But judging from published reports and informal talk, anthropologists in applied settings are often preoccupied with proving themselves as competent in someone else's terms—as capable of being a good sociologist, a good public-health scientist, a good evaluation specialist, a good health educator. In these situations, our native professional voices, and our capacities for self-reflection, may be obscured. This may rebound on us, constraining our development as anthropologists, changing our affiliation to our home discipline, and causing us to question whether we can describe what we do as anthropology. Thus, a critical anthropology *of* applied settings, as distinct from a critical anthropology *in* applied settings, is not accomplished often enough (cf. Johannsen 1992).

In the chapters to follow, I will trace a debate about cancer causation and connect this debate to deeper conflicts concerning power, truth, and meaning. Throughout, I will look at my own role, the role of the anthropologist, and at how I myself lived the conflicts I explore. Tannerstown has declined to serve as my beginning point. We are as good as they are, say the people of Tannerstown, so do not make *us* the object of your study. In attempting to take this advice, I shift to a more critical perspective on the professional cultures I saw and experienced. Thus, in a sense, my own discomfort about the conflicts I lived becomes my beginning point.

I still carry the siren song of acceptance by the medical community as a strong internal voice. I am afraid that my work will be taken to imply that the recommendations of scientific cancer control do not constitute good advice. I do not mean to imply that. I do want to support people who are trying to quit smoking and to encourage people to ask their physicians about getting cancer tests. But such advice is not given in a vacuum. The social and cultural context in which it is formulated, transmitted, and interpreted is built of professional authorities; tensions between social classes; ideologies of inequality, legitimacy, blame, and sickness; and moral images of what it means to live a healthy life. It is my purpose to describe this context and to question whether it is an appropriate and fruitful context for the practice of health education. As I pursue this question, my fear of disapproval from my former colleagues keeps arising. I hope that this fear has not constrained my thinking in unimagined ways.

THE STUDY COMMUNITY | 2

It is the food we eat, the alcohol we drink, and the tobacco we smoke or otherwise abuse that, more than any other factors, have increased our risk of cancer. The enemy is not the chemical plant down the street, but ourselves.

J. W. Yarbro, "Carcinogenesis," in *Cancer Nursing: Principles and Practice,* ed. Susan L. Groenwald and others

I think we live in a high-risk area, being with all the chemical plants and all. I know a lot of my neighbors have died from cancer. It's a scary thing. . . . In this neighborhood, that's all you hear.

Tannerstown resident

The community served by the cancer-control project on which I worked is actually a series of small, socially cohesive neighborhoods, geographically contiguous and socially and physically similar. Tannerstown is one of these neighborhoods, the one in which most of my own work was done and the bulk of my data collected.

A BRIEF HISTORY

Tannerstown has been a European-American working-class community since colonial times.[1] When early settlers in Philadelphia complained of noxious odors from certain types of enterprises—notably tanning and fishing—these enterprises moved up the Delaware River, north of the city. With them moved their workers, who built small towns around their sources of employment. Through the years, Philadelphia grew out to incorporate these small towns, and then grew way past them. Tannerstown and other former small towns are now part of Philadelphia's inner city. The general area of Philadelphia in which Tannerstown is located is today variously known as Greater Kensington, the old Lower Northeast, or, most colorfully, the river wards.

Following World War I, at a time of expansion in industrial chemical production, Tannerstown enjoyed a period of great growth. Modern chemical plants were built adjacent to the community, and additional workers settled nearby. Together, the three largest chemical plants, and the support industries that grew up around them, employed a high percentage of local residents. The "Big Three" companies enjoyed a paternalistic relationship with Tannerstown and other nearby communities—there were softball leagues, Christmas baskets for the needy, yearly picnics at company expense, and donations to community causes. At the plants, family and long-time friends worked together.

The river wards chemical plants fared well throughout the 1950s, benefiting from the post–World War II boom in chemicals production. As industry in the United States declined in the decades that followed, however, the neighborhoods in the river wards did not fare well. One of the Big Three closed down—as did other large river wards employers. Unemployment in the river wards rose, the population of the neighborhoods aged, and a major interstate highway cut through the area. At the same time, residents of the river wards, along with the rest of the country, began to raise serious questions about the health risks of exposure to industrial chemicals and to air pollution from industry and heavy street traffic. Today, in short, Tannerstown still lives with industrial pollution that no one else wants—but the advantages and the perceived advantages of doing so have diminished.

Data from the U.S. Bureau of the Census point to Tannerstown today as a small, stable working-class neighborhood (Table 1). At the 1990 census, the population of Tannerstown was counted as 6,531, the neighborhood's population decline mirroring that of Philadelphia as a whole. The age distribution for Tannerstown is not dramatically different from that for the entire city, although Tannerstown does have a higher percentage of residents age fifty-five to eighty-four years old. The median value of a Tannerstown house is about the same as for the city as a whole. Vacancy rates are lower, rates of home ownership are higher, and a greater percentage of occupants have been in their homes since 1959 or earlier. Data from the 1980 census indicate that in Tannerstown, as compared with all Philadelphia, a far higher percent-

Table 1. Description of the Population of Tannerstown, Compared with That of Philadelphia County (City of Philadelphia)

	Tannerstown[a]	Philadelphia
Population Characteristics		
Total population	6,531	1,585,577
Population decline, 1970–90	15.8%	18.6%
Median age	36.6	33.2
European-American	99.3%	53.5%
Housing Characteristics		
Total housing units	2,593	674,899
Median value, all units	$45,382	$49,369
Vacancy rates, year-round, all units	2.9%	6.5%
Units build 1959 or earlier	96.3%	79.3%
Occupant in unit since 1959 or earlier	34.5%	16.5%
Owner-occupied, of occupied units	84.2%	55.4%
Indicators of Socioeconomic Status		
Education		
High school graduates, age 25+	32.3%	32.9%
College graduates, age 25+	3.7%	8.9%
Students in private elementary/high school	49.5%	29.2%
Occupation		
Professional, technical, manager, proprietor	21.0%	28.6%
Clerical	25.8%	21.8%
Sales	9.1%	9.7%
Crafts	13.6%	9.0%
Operators, laborers	20.0%	14.1%
Service	10.5%	16.3%
Income		
Median household income	$27,539	$24,603
Unemployment rate, civilian	5.3%	9.6%

Sources: All data are drawn from United States census figures. Data for 1990 were compiled by Urban Decision Systems, Inc. (1992). Data for 1970, used with data from the above referenced source to calculate "Population decline," are from U.S. Bureau of the Census 1972, Table P-1.

a. Some figures for Tannerstown represent a weighted average of figures from two census tracts. The figure for unemployment also represents a weighted average between female and male unemployment rates.

age of owner-occupied units are owned without a mortgage (70.2 percent and 50.2 percent, respectively [U.S. Bureau of the Census 1983]).

Indicators of socioeconomic status also point to Tannerstown as a modest but stable neighborhood. Compared with all Philadelphians, a lower percentage of Tannerstowners have graduated from college. As recently as 1980, Tannerstowners were also less likely than all Philadelphians to have graduated from high school (U.S. Bureau of the Census 1983); data from the 1990 census indicate, however, that rates of high school graduation have remained steady in Tannerstown while they have fallen in other areas of the city. A very high percentage of Tannerstown families pay to send their children to private (mostly Catholic) schools. Tannerstowners are less likely to hold professional and managerial jobs, and more likely to work in crafts or as operators or laborers; these patterns are less pronounced, however, than they were at the 1980 census. Median household income is similar to that for the city as whole, with similar distributions. At the 1980 census, there was a lower percentage of families living below the poverty level in Tannerstown than in the city as a whole (U.S. Bureau of the Census 1983). Data do show that Tannerstowners, with the rest of those in the river wards, are among the poorest of European-American Philadelphians.[2] All in all, however, these data indicate that Tannerstown is an economically modest but successful neighborhood.

Despite economic stresses—shared by many in the United States—Tannerstown is, in fact, one of the more stable communities of the river wards. Tannerstown feels like a small, tightly knit industrial town. Most of the houses are old and faced with brick or stone, which projects a feeling of many years of meticulous care. Lines of small rowhouses are interspersed with single and double houses, some with yards and pretty gardens. It is common for Tannerstown families to have roots in the neighborhood that go back three or four generations. Many Tannerstowners seldom leave their neighborhood and have limited experience with outside agencies. The social lives of most residents revolve around family, neighborhood, and church. The area is heavily Catholic, with both geographic and ethnic parishes, and most neighborhood children attend Catholic schools. The tall spires of the various Catholic churches are visible everywhere and serve to orient resident and visitor alike. The neighborhood feels self-contained: streets are narrow and well worn, everyone knows the same people, and few come in or leave without being noticed.

The air in Tannerstown has a distinctive odor. It is one of the first things an outsider notices. It is a dusty smell with an acrid undertone, something like the stale air of an old high school chemistry laboratory. On days when the smell was particularly strong, I used to joke to myself that it might clear my sinuses. But it can smell that way and be a beautiful day in Tannerstown. Smell or no smell, Tannerstown is a great place to walk, a place to feel a sense of belonging, a real face-to-face community.

Most Tannerstowners trace the odor to air pollution from the large chemical plants in the area. Near those plants, this pollution leaves constant reminders: the ever-present odor; a white film on the windowsills; and billowing smokestacks that, some residents claim, are especially active on the weekends, when the local office of the Environmental Protection Agency is closed (see Figure 1).

THE "CANCER HOT SPOT"

Tannerstown is a high-cancer-risk area. As an inner-city neighborhood in Philadelphia, one would expect it to be. Nationally, cancer mortality is higher in cities than it is in rural areas, and it is higher in the Northeast than in other areas of the country. Philadelphia is within an area of particularly high cancer incidence. But even accounting for all this, the river wards area of the city has a higher rate than would be expected (Dayal et al. 1984).[3]

One of the enduring questions about areas of high cancer risk—called cancer clusters, or cancer "hot spots"—is whether they are linked to pollution of the nonoccupational environment. It seems clear that certain cancers, including some lung cancers, are linked to certain exposures common in occupational settings (such as mesothelioma to asbestos). It is less clear whether one's cancer risk is increased if one

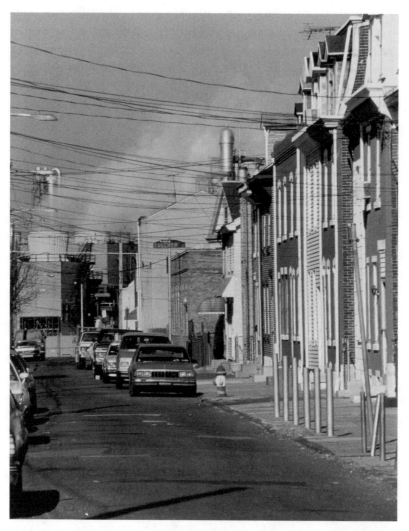

Figure 1. Tannerstown on a Saturday morning. Photograph by Howard Balshem.

lives in an area of high ambient air pollution, such as may be caused by oil refineries, chemical companies, or heavy concentrations of automobile exhaust. Several lines of research provide indirect support for the suggestion that the link between air pollution and cancer risk is real.[4] The research questions involved are complex, however. First, in any given case of cancer, many factors may have been contributory. This is especially true for cases in which cancer develops over a long period of time—a common circumstance in carcinogenesis. Second, air pollution, even if implicated in cancer causation, may cause only a small, difficult-to-detect number of excess cases. Third, for many cancers, not enough is known about how the disease develops to speculate knowledgeably about how air pollutants might act in carcinogenesis. Fourth, the sensibilities of some cancer researchers seem to draw from a possibly accurate political awareness that industrial nations are basically unwilling to reduce their dependence on synthetic materials and fossil fuels, even if this dependence means an increased risk of cancer among some population subgroups. Because of all this, polluters can state that there is no research that clearly shows a link between cancer and air pollution and, furthermore, can cite plenty of published material that takes a very conservative, even negative view of the research that does suggest such a link.

Most studies that are done on the topic are based on ecologic analysis. Such analyses are based on comparisons of the patterns of geographical distribution for different variables. It is a correlational methodology: one can see if variables are distributed in similar fashion, but not whether they are causally related. Dayal et al. (1984) present an ecologic analysis of correlates to cancer mortality rates in Philadelphia. Using data compiled by census tract, Dayal and his coworkers looked for differences by neighborhood. Their analysis indicated that areas with high cancer mortality also exhibit low socioeconomic status and that high lung cancer mortality among men is distributed with high air pollution (sulfur dioxide and total suspended particulates). Because lung cancer (and total cancer) among women does not exhibit the same clustering, the researchers discount the possibility that air pollution alone could be causing the high lung cancer rates among men. They suggest that smoking and exposure to toxins in the workplace— risk factors that correlate with socioeconomic status—explain the high cancer rates for men in certain neighborhoods, and that women are not as strongly affected because fewer of them smoke or work with industrial chemicals. The authors point to the possibility, however, of a more complex role for air pollution, perhaps through a synergism with smoking. They carefully acknowledge the limitations of their analysis.

The Dayal study is fairly well known in the river wards. At public functions, residents sometimes questioned me, usually sharply, about the study. By and large, they downplayed or ignored the researchers' careful caveats, and spoke of the article as a denial, by scientists, of the link between cancer and air pollution. To the extent that Tanners-towners connect their high cancer rates to industrial pollution, this scientific denial was bitterly derided. The following quotation is from a woman in her thirties, a resident of a river wards neighborhood near Tannerstown; she weaves her awareness of the Dayal study into a general picture of resentment toward scientific experts:

I mean, you know, they've narrowed it down today but they're not real sure. Then they say—I mean we've asked—you know, the people in this area—and they say, "well, could be the environment that we live in, that's why women get it and men get it but the women aren't going into the work place and that has to be the air that you're breathing." You know. Or, you know, "And then you have smoking, you get it from smoking." But then you have somebody dies of cancer who's never smoked a ciga-rette in their lives. So, you know, so I mean there's just so *many* things I think that lead to cancer and I don't think scientists have narrowed it down enough yet.

Tannerstown may be described, through reference to data on cancer morbidity and mortality, as a cancer hot spot. It is also a community in which cancer is an important internal concern. As we shall see next, high cancer rates are also a key element of the community's image in the wider metropolitan area.

IMAGES OF TANNERSTOWN

Philadelphians are fond of describing their city as a "city of neighbor-hoods." Many working-class people, especially minorities, still live in the old, inner-city neighborhoods. Most who have moved out are proud to trace their family's roots back to one of the older, working-class areas of the city. The old neighborhoods are remembered fondly. The common memory is of large families squeezed into small row houses, extended family in other row houses near by, and all the neighbors visiting out on the front stoop. Younger people in Philadelphia who still live in some of these neighborhoods—notably, the Italian areas of South Philadelphia—enjoy a certain prestige, reflecting Philadelphia's self-concept, accurate or not, as a working-class city and the desire of many Philadelphians to claim economically modest roots.

If Philadelphia celebrates the old working-class neighborhood, the various neighborhoods of the river wards ought to qualify for high prestige. Many Philadelphians, however, see the river wards as an area they love to hate. The neighborhoods are known as tough and dirty, and negative images of area residents abound. "Those people down there," I once heard a lifelong Philadelphian say, "are the scum of the earth." "Oh, lovely area to be working in," another acquaintance said sarcastically when I told her I was working on a project in the river wards. Both of these people are themselves from modest social backgrounds, the second from a poor working-class area.

In reality, the river wards are variegated; some areas are settled and even prosperous and some are run-down, with many abandoned houses. Some neighborhoods in the area lend themselves well to being romanticized as old face-to-face communities, whereas others are more easily demonized as examples of urban decay. In part, it depends on where you look, both geographically and metaphorically. Two photographs (Figure 2) illustrate the range of images that represent the area. Both were taken for use in slide presentations for professional groups concerned with health programs in the community. Both are accurate in that they represent sights commonly seen in the river wards. The first picture, which shows the backs of houses and trash in close detail, was taken by a health professional who lives in the river wards and is a native of another working-class neighborhood in the city. The photograph was used to illustrate a talk on the extreme difficulties of doing health education work in the area. The second picture was taken to illustrate an oral presentation of my own on the value of community solidarity in one of the river wards neighborhoods, which together were described as having a Dickensian feeling. Both images were created to speak to a central contention among

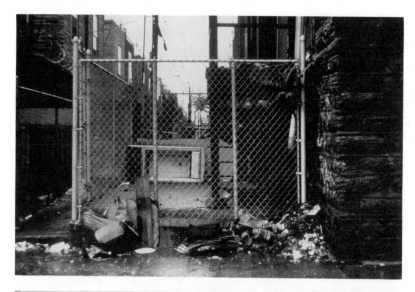

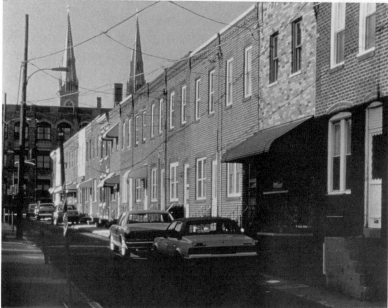

Figure 2. Two images of the river wards. *Top:* Trash in a back alley. Photograph by Joan James. *Bottom:* Rowhouses and church spires. Photograph by Howard Balshem.

those who construct images of the river wards. The first image says that toughness, dirt, and decay are at the center of why it is hard to do community health education in the river wards. The second says that there is a solid heart and soul in the center of the area's life. These views are not necessarily contradictory, but their counterposition motivated the design of both of these photographic images.

Mass-media images of the river wards show a similarly strong contrast. Such images are particularly clear in three publications: the *Philadelphia Daily News,* which is the local working-class tabloid; *Philadelphia Magazine,* which is a glossy, pricey magazine for the upscale baby-boomer; and the *Guide,* a community newspaper for the river wards. In all three publications, references to high cancer rates, and to the ways that river wards residents respond to them, help to build the general image of the area.

"The Cancer Zones"

In 1981 the *Philadelphia Daily News* published a five-part series entitled "The Cancer Zones." This series reported a *Daily News* investigation of areas in the Philadelphia region that had higher rates of cancer mortality than would be expected. The investigation was a collaboration between the *Daily News* and the Philadelphia city health department, and involved four months of research in the "cancer zone" communities by a *Daily News* reporter, Juan Gonzalez. The series opens with a front-page headline reading "Cancer Death Zones: Probe Pinpoints City Hot Spots" and continues on another page with the headline: "Cancer Hot Spots: Fatalities Rampant in 2 Neighborhoods." One of the hot spots identified includes Tannerstown.

The series has the flavor of an exposé. On January 5, the first day of the series, an introductory article states that the investigation was impeded by the absence of a statewide tumor registry (since established), and by the failure of the city health department to study the problem. In this article, the *Daily News* investigation is described as the first of its kind attempted. This is held to be an especially grievous oversight, because Philadelphia has such high cancer rates.

The series takes a definite environmentalist stance, strongly suggesting that high cancer rates in certain areas can be traced to industrial pollution. Lifestyle theories of cancer causation are given short shrift and made to look unfair. As discussed earlier, lifestyle theories of disease tend to draw from constructions of sick or high-risk people as foolish, morally flawed, or ignorant. But the people in the Cancer Zones series are carefully portrayed counter to this construction. They are portrayed as hard-working people who often gave long years of faithful service to the industries that poisoned them; as family people with long roots in their neighborhoods; and as people who are deservedly angry and willing to stand up and say that they were poisoned. The following portrait of one resident of a high-cancer-risk area, drawn in an article by Juan Gonzalez published on January 8, 1981, illustrates much of this:

For 67 years, Mary Caselli's life has revolved around the mill. Starting during the Depression, she gave the best of her years to the textile division of [a] giant asbestos plant in [her town]. . . . "Everybody's worked there," says Caselli of [her] townspeople. Her niece, Carla DiScala, who only worked a few years in the plant, gave it the most—her life. On St. Patrick's Day in 1973, Carla died at age 53 of mesothelioma, a rare lung disease almost always caused by exposure to asbestos. . . .

Carla had worked as a spinner in Plant 4, textile division, for only a few years . . . But throughout her life, her aunt says, Carla slept in the second-floor front bedroom of Caselli's home, which was exposed to the worst of the asbestos dust released from the plant.

"Sometimes it (the dust) was so bad you could wipe it like a film off the window and the furniture," Caselli said. "One night, I called the plant manager in the middle of the night. It got so bad I had trouble breathing. I told him, "If I can't sleep at night, you're not sleeping either unless you do something about that dust." She says that soon after, the plant got a new dust collector on its stacks. . . .

A spokesman for the state Department of Environmental Resources said recent testing of the air outside [the plant] showed no abnormal asbestos levels . . . . Anger and frustration swell in Caselli's eyes. . . . "It's bad," she says of company resistance. "They won't admit it's ever asbestosis because the more they pay out, the more their insurance goes up." Caselli's mother used to work in the sewing department, making fireman's gloves and suits. Caselli says her mother told her that sometimes the workers were ankle-deep in piles of asbestos dust. "But each time they (the company) got wind of someone from the state or the government coming, we had to practically lick the machines clean for inspection. They were slick that way," Caselli says.

Mary Caselli's life has revolved around the mill, but this has dampened neither her willingness to speak out against the mill owners nor her perception that they have no regard for the health of those who work in and live around the mill. She owns a dramatic history, marked by personal tragedy, and she remains resolved and self-possessed. She is explicitly drawn, through the details we are given, as *not* foolish, morally flawed, or ignorant. In fact, like several other characters drawn in the Cancer Zones series, she has long suspected her risks. Years ago, the *Daily News* discourse goes, residents of these high-risk communities did not give much thought to cancer, but they grew to suspect their health risks long before anything official was published. The Cancer Zones series reads as a vindication of their suspicions. These good people have been victimized by disinformation from the industries and by the inaction of public officials sworn to work for the protection of the public health. According to the *Daily News*, residents of the Cancer Zones may be victims, but they are perceptive ones.

These community residents are counterposed in the *Daily News* series to spokespersons for industry and government. Spokespersons for industry are quoted as consistently denying problems or as saying that pollution problems existed in the past but are now solved. They are often drawn as irate. Public officials are made to look surprised by the information uncovered by the *Daily News*. They are made to seem slightly bewildered and generally inept. The basic picture is that they have essentially been caught asleep at the wheel. The following, excerpted from an article by Juan Gonzalez on January 5, is illustrative:

[H]ealth officials apparently weren't aware of the high death rates in the . . . communities until now, because the health department has never studied cancer figures city-wide and because the state does not require central registration of cancer tumors. When told of the *Daily News* findings, City Health Commissioner Lewis Polk said: "It certainly warrants looking into. We would be interested in reviewing the material to see what might be our logical next step."

. . . Former [river wards] resident Kitty Mack, whose own bout with cancer has led her to a career in environmental law, thinks the figures warrant a full-scale investigation. Mack . . . considers herself one of [the] "lucky" ones—even though doctors say chances are 3 in 10 the brain tumor for which she was operated on last year will return. "There wasn't much publicity about toxic chemicals then," said Mack, 29, as she recalled the "dust and the smell" that was part of her youth in [the river wards]. . . . Of her experiences with cancer, she says: "It was horrible. I felt very angry. And the more I see and read about how cancer is caused by the environment, the angrier I get. Nobody should have to go through what I went through at age 28." Response to the *Daily News* investigation from spokesmen for plants in the hot spot areas was mixed. "We know of no health effects associated with discharges from our [plant]," [a chemical company spokesperson] told the *Daily News*. . . . "Twenty or 30 years ago, downtown Philadelphia was covered with coal ash. Downtown Pittsburgh was a disaster area. It's a long time away in the history of where industry has moved in this country. Why bring it up?" said [a spokesperson for an oil company], whose 100,000-barrel-a-day refinery borders the portion of South Philadelphia that ranks as the city's No. 1 hot spot.

Again, the community resident quoted is explicitly *not* foolish, morally flawed, or ignorant. The contrast between her and the industry spokespersons is emotionally effective, tapping the reader's presumedly established anger at and disdain for powerful industrial interests.

The *Philadelphia Daily News* is written for working-class readers. In the case of the Cancer Zones series, as in much *Daily News* writing, the underlying discourse is one of familiarity between the readers and the lay people represented in the text. This is perhaps most dramatically experienced through the photographs that accompany the articles. One image, published on January 7, shows a long-time resident of one high-risk neighborhood sitting at a table at the small local restaurant she owns: she leans forward, a pleasant face with a friendly, open expression, and a cup of coffee in her hand. The perspective of the photographer encourages readers to imagine themselves sitting across the table from her. Another photograph, printed two days later, shows the face of a man whose wife died at the age of forty-two from cancer. The article implicates a workplace hazard—a microfilm copier housed with inadequate ventilation in Philadelphia's City Hall, which had not been removed even after it had been shown to emit high levels of ozone. In the photograph, the widower's face is shown in the bottom quarter, grim with unresolved anger, teeth clenched with the pain of thinking about it, even years later. City Hall tower dominates the rest of the picture, looming like a monolith in the background, a seemingly unassailable authority. Again, there is easy emotional resonance between the reader and the unfortunate man in the photograph.

The image of the resident of the cancer hot spot—or, as in the last example, the victim of workplace hazards—is a proud image of the working class: honestly willing to live in obedience to industrial labor but independent and perceptive about the abuses that characterize the exercise of power by industry and government. The hot-spot residents who were quoted may not know a lot about cancer science, but they surely know more than the public health officials do. This discourse about common people runs counter to the discourse that underlies lifestyle theories of cancer causation. It states that common people are morally decent and clear-sighted and that public officials and captains of industry are not. It states that common people make clear rational sense and possess moral independence from knowledge generated by powerful interests. Officially legitimate knowledge is presented as full of convenient holes, as created in the service of industry, and as therefore morally corrupt. Residents of polluted communities—or workers in hazardous workplaces—are morally sound partly *because* they represent a resistance to receipt of this knowledge. Their resistance is born of perception, not ignorance. They may smoke or eat the wrong things, but they are solid people, and their insights into the power structures they live with are normal, honest, familiar, and fair. They are valorized as morally undefeated.

"The New White Ghetto"

A very different image is presented in *Philadelphia Magazine*. This image is presented not in a formal series but in occasional articles that feature images of the river wards. Two important such articles were written by Mike Mallowe, a local journalist. Directly and indirectly,

Mallowe refers to Peter Binzen's *Whitetown USA* (Binzen 1970). In the *Philadelphia Magazine* articles, as in Binzen's book, life in the river wards is presented as dominated by the gloom of urban decay. The streets are tough, filthy, and dangerous, the local elevated transit line is rusting and falling apart, and the people are bitter, ill-tempered, and narrow-minded, trapped inside what Mallowe calls "the spell of the Kensington state of mind" (1979:245). To lead off one article, Mallowe describes a night spent driving around one river wards neighborhood with a local resident. They drive by a local bar and see kids hanging out on the corner. "The kids must have known the old man I was with because as our car approached, they faded back into the darkness near the taproom's brick walls. Everybody but her. She stood her ground and stared right into my window on the passenger's side. She started to giggle, turned and said something to the kids behind her, then lifted the quart in the brown paper bag and chugged it like a champ. She couldn't have been more than 10 years old" (Mallowe 1979:89). This is a romantic image of a sort, presented with a brooding, self-conscious cadence. It is an image of the urban wasteland. Urban decay is illustrated for the reader not only through descriptions of inanimate objects—decaying El girders, iron grating on store windows—but also through descriptions of the people: "The kids with beer, the kids who strip cars, the kids who break windows, the kids who set fire to vacant buildings, the kids who buy pills with nickels and dimes, the kids who sniff glue, the kids who use school yards as urinals, the kids who throw anything they can lift at the El trains, the kids who assault old people, the kids who gather 15- and 20-strong on the street corners, and the kids who, according to the lifetime residents, give the neighborhood a bad name, fall between the law enforcement cracks in Whitetown" (Mallowe 1979:92).

Adult residents of the river wards do not fare much better. They have "always voted from emotion, not reason" (Mallowe 1979:242). They resist a new public high school in their area because they fear the encroachment of minorities: "And so an entire section of the city has been willing to self-destructively deny its teenage boys a modern, functioning public high school, opting instead for a drop-out rate as bad as or worse than any non-white neighborhood in the city" (Mallowe 1979:244–45).

In a later article, Mallowe blames social decay in the river wards and similar areas on the loss of blue-collar manufacturing jobs. But his focus is still clearly on urban decay and on the people as part of what has decayed in the river wards. He constructs a strong view of the state of mind of people who live in what he calls "the new white ghetto":

You are poor, or close to it; white; able to read just well enough to get by; existing in a dying landscape of closed factories, blue-collar jobs that no longer exist, streets that mark racial boundaries as effectively as the Berlin Wall, and church, school and government programs that touch your life not at all.

You represent a hefty percentage—maybe as much as 30 percent—of the 900,000 white people who still live in Philadelphia. You aren't going anywhere. You need a job to make it in the suburbs, but the only jobs you can handle are the kind that used to keep the families in the neighborhood together. All those jobs are gone now. So are the strong unions and the sense of immigrant cohesion that once made your grandparents so secure. Now, all you have is yourself, and that doesn't seem to count for much anymore.

Other *Philadelphia Magazine* images of the poor European-American working class make less of an attempt to be analytical and simply play social-class stereotypes for laughs. A clear example of this is the occasional series entitled "Philadelphia Style." This series presents a tongue-in-cheek view of eight communities in the Philadelphia area—seven city neighborhoods and one suburb—through caricatures of supposedly typical residents. No one is spared. The residents of all eight neighborhoods are made to look ridiculous. The humor is derisive, mocking, and cynical. Fishtown, which is a river wards neighborhood, is used to represent the bottom of the socioeconomic barrel. Material drawn from this series is presented in Table 2.

In these sardonic images of social class, the relationship between image and reader is not one of easy identity, as it is for the working-class reader of the *Daily News*. The Philadelphia Style stereotypes are drawn to appeal to readers who see themselves as déclassé intellec-

Table 2. Two Social-Class Caricatures in *Philadelphia Magazine*

	Chestnut Hill Prep	Fishtown Fundamental
Philadelphia Style		
DRESS	Navy blazer, loud plaid slacks, bow tie, khakis . . .	Steel-toed work shoes, tractor cap, Sears work pants . . .
CAR	1976 Volvo	Chevy van with body cancer
LAST BOOK READ	Book-of-the-Month Club Alternate Selection	Baltimore Catechism
BUMPER STICKER	"I Brake for Animals"	"Roofers Need Love, Too"
RELIGION	You really have to ask?	Anti-Semitism
A Philadelphia-style Christmas		
HOW TO SPEND THE HOLIDAYS	At home, feeling superior	Blitzed
FAVORITE HOLIDAY DRINK	Hot toddy in the library	A six-pack
WHO PLAYS SANTA	The butler	Big Sid from the taproom
Philadelphia Style Goes to the Shore		
LAST THING TO DO BEFORE LEAVING HOME	Take the golden retriever to the kennel	Lock the dog in the basement
BEACH BAG	L. L. Bean canvas boat tote	Plastic Amway bag
FAVORITE SEAFOOD DINNER	Clambake with Maine lobster	Chicken of the Sea
Tying the Knot Philly Style		
INVITATION	Caldwell's standard	Xeroxed
WHAT TO SERVE	Korbel champagne and enough tea sandwiches so each guest gets one . . .	Schmidt's and Ball Park franks
ATTIRE	Courtney wears Great-grandmother Darlington's lace gown . . .	Diane wears her mother's wedding dress, of course. From the maternity department at Sears . . .

Sources: Saline et al. 1981; Saline and the Philadelphia Magazine staff 1981; Gale et al. 1982; Kitei 1984.

tuals, and social-class identity as something ugly and ridiculous. The more serious *Philadelphia Magazine* articles about working-class life function to keep readers feeling well-informed, essential for those who feel that mental acuity removes them from the class system. The parallel humor pieces are deliciously funny to people who feel that their intellect permits them to laugh at everyone. Obviously, the self-declared déclassé intellectual is acutely aware of social class. Both the serious and humorous articles discussed here support this awareness, assuring readers that they are informed in depth about the social-class system but are excused from participation in it because of cynicism.[5]

With regard to the river wards, the summary *Philadelphia Magazine* image is urban decay, decay that is located partially in the people. This is the mechanism that is at the root of the blame-the-victim stance. The image presented suggests despair to be the knowledgeable stance toward social problems in the river wards. But fun can be had in the meantime: the upscale and their allies can be in the know about the colorful folks at the bottom of the social scale. The lives of these folks are described through a focus on disease, decay, and disintegration— an urban cancer, a social cancer, an area and a people beyond the regulation of the normal body politic.

The high cancer rates and poor general health suffered by river wards residents are fit into this general picture. The author of one *Philadelphia Magazine* article (Duffy 1982) talks about community resistance to industrial polluters in one river wards neighborhood, describing the neighborhood as divided and confused by the struggle against the firms that have employed them. Mallowe paints a bleak portrait of the health lifestyles said to be typical of the area—smoking, drinking, illicit drugs, morbid obesity, teen pregnancy, poor prenatal care—and quotes a physician at a river wards hospital as stating: "This is a cancer corridor and half of it is self-induced" (Mallowe 1986:168). In this article, the river wards are described as a health war zone, and the war is described as being fought between the dedicated health professionals who work in the area and the ignorant and indifferent residents. In the following excerpt, a nun working in the river wards hospital describes a pregnant teenage woman who has taken illicit drugs shortly before going into labor:

"[H]ere she is ready to deliver this baby and she's swallowing this junk! How does anybody get through to them?" Still, Sister [W] continues to try. She looks away, distracted, trembling from anger and frustration. The silence in the dark room now begs a vexing question: Exactly *whom* should you be mad at? The kids? The pushers? The neighborhood? The economic factors, faceless and elusive, that have combined, conspired, to sap the life of this once-thriving community—sap it more each day with the departure of each additional manufacturing or craft or machinist's job? "I'll have to be going now," Sister [W] says resignedly. "You asked what it was like. Now you know." (Mallowe 1986:169)

The "you" who asked what it was like, and who cannot decide at whom to be angry, is as much the reader as it is the writer. What Mallowe tells the reader, through the authority of Sister W., is that there are no answers and that the people of the river wards will not cooperate in their own salvation. This absolves the reader from all obligation, even from the effort to understand.

"By Dan"

A third media image of life in the river wards is found in the popular column "by Dan," which appears in the *Guide*. "By Dan" is a gossip and social commentary column, featuring letters and other reports of community goings-on, as reported by residents of the neighborhoods. These reports are annotated by Dan's commentary. The voices in the column, including Dan's, are directed internally, toward public opinion in the river wards.

The "by Dan" column is very popular in Tannerstown and other river wards neighborhoods. A review of forty of the columns, printed from January 18, 1979, to August 18, 1988, in various editions of the *Guide*, reveals several dominating themes.[6]

First among these is criticism or ridicule of area residents for stepping out of neighborhood social norms. People are called to task for being insincere, unfriendly, superior, stingy, or just different. The following passages illustrate this. As here, initials for street and personal names are used in the original columns.

'ROUND THE AREA: We can't understand how HR of "E" St. can walk around with that mop of hair. We know he's no great spender but when you need a haircut, you need one, as your head looks sloppy with hair in an untidy fashion. . . . Would you believe that GC of "F" St. constantly rips girls who walk around with lo-cut tops—and then she goes out and rents a porno video? You have to be consistent, my dear.

SOURPUSS: How about BG of "A" St. and her sour disposition? It's hard to fathom how an individual can go through life with such unhappiness. Whose fault is it that she has no male companions? Whose fault is it that she stays home with her mother all the time instead of going out to meet guys? No one's fault but her own. So why does she take it out on her neighbors, asks CK, who lives near the gal. BG never smiles. She often looks the other way when her neighbors come out of their house. If she's working on her car or doing something outside her house she offers no recognition when neighbors appear. She's just a loner and she likely will remain that way unless she changes her attitude. But we have little hope she will.

QUESTIONS OF THE WEEK: . . . Wouldn't it be better if VP of "W" St. placed her mother in a nursing home rather than have her so uncomfortable at home? We know it costs money, but VP should think of the well-being of her mother rather than her purse strings.[7]

The "by Dan" image of the typical river wards resident—based on passages such as these and on other, more positive passages—is of someone who is generous, sociable, caring toward family and neighbors, and self-sacrificing. The author of "by Dan" is merciless toward those who fail to live up to this image, presenting river wards people as demanding, and being used to, a certain level of decency among neighbors. In these tightly knit neighborhoods, refusing to socialize or share resources are notable transgressions.

Another dominant theme, closely related to the first, is that of maintaining accepted standards for the external appearance of one's house. Constance Perin (1988) offers a discussion of neighborly relations in middle-class suburbs that is strikingly similar. As in Perin's discussion, there are two main types of complaints against neighbors: one, they fail to maintain their own property; and two, they invade the property of others in various ways, such as by letting their dogs wander.

HERE AND THERE: . . . If HA of "D" St. ever cleaned his sidewalk when it snowed it would be a miracle. He just let folks slide and slip on his front during the recent bad weather and didn't give a darn. His neighbors were hoping that he would be the one to fall on his fanny.[8]

Well, the dog problems are with us again. Take this note from EB of "C" St.: "Kensington has had Clean Up and Feel Proud days. Could you please have a 'Keep Your Dog In Your Own Yard Day?' I have cleaned up at one time seven or eight 'gifts' left by dogs in the alley beside my house and my pavement. . . . Our main offender is a large Doberman. I try not to annoy my neighbors, so does anyone know why I'm being annoyed? Maybe someone can write a column to curb 'pet owners.' " Well, this problem is a continuing one and one for which we don't have a solution. . . . If there is only one Doberman at fault, why don't you dump all the doo-doo on that neighbor's pavement or front steps to let the owner know you know who's doing it.[9]

Dan offers his readers more than a simple statement of social transgression. He also takes the perpetrator down a peg. His style of humor is burlesque: the reader laughs in glee at the image of the inconsiderate neighbor falling on his fanny, or stepping out the front door into a pile of dog doo-doo. The central message is what it always is in burlesque: don't be so high and mighty; come down to the same level as the rest of us.

A third major theme in "by Dan" is romance, an ever-popular topic here as elsewhere. In "by Dan," the foibles of people in the throes of romance or passion are usually played for laughs. People have a long lead before they are considered to have gone into the realm of the truly offensive. Up until that point, they are just considered funny.

WIFE'S AWAY: KL of "L" St. writes: "RP of "A" St. thinks he's pulling a fast one, but we are all on to him. His wife and children are vacationing at her mother's house for several weeks and RP goes down on the weekends.

But he's not sleeping alone at home during the week for his next door neighbor saw a woman sneak into the back door the other night. The neighbor was ready to call the police because of all the noise but she decided to listen through the wall, and she had almost as much fun as they did. Somebody was chasing somebody up and down the steps and then there would be silence for about an hour. Then it started all over again. RP's wife is going to start wondering why he's so tired when he comes down for the weekend. I can't blame him, because she's no angel and we all know why they got married in the first place."

It's not often the man is the chasee and the woman is the chaser but that is the case of SZ and AB as evidenced by this letter from SZ: "Whatya going to do when a woman is after you and you are only attracted to her by her money and her connections? That's my problem with a lady (AB) who is pursuing me constantly. . . . We sit next to each other at Flyers games but that's because she owns the tickets and graciously sells me one. . . . I value her friendship but it's getting more difficult all the time to stave her off." Some guys would love your problem, especially since the gal is so well fixed. . . . We know she is no raving beauty, having seen her, so we can see your point. But we've seen you too, and you're far from Paul Newman yourself. . . . you have your choice—break it off altogether and possibly forfeit your chance to get Flyer tickets next season or try her once and see what she or you are missing.[10]

PRACTICE MAKES PERFECT: We heard that WD and SM of "F" St. are going to tie the knot. Everyone thought they were living in wedded bliss but they were just practicing for the real thing.[11]

QUESTION OF THE WEEK: Who did HB of "K" St. go across to Jersey with two Saturday nights ago? That wasn't her regular boy friend and that motel wasn't her house.[12]

In "by Dan," people are displayed as being slightly ridiculous when in the pursuit of romance. The courtship displays of one's neighbors are as amusing as those on a TV nature show. The reader is cautioned, however, not to fall into a superior attitude. Listening to the moral transgressions of others is good, clean fun, but the reader has no right to criticize unless he or she is without sin—which, if the truth be known, hardly anybody is.

In addition to romance and community standards for behavior, "by

Dan" takes up another important theme: complaints about government services and municipal authorities. These complaints focus most strongly on services that touch people's daily lives: postal carriers, city police, city sanitation workers, public school teachers, and welfare cheaters. The following quotations are typical:

"I love to read your column and now I am writing you to let you know how I feel about the stamp going up. We get bad service and the only time it is good is when the regular mailmen are on duty. When the other mailmen are on, we get the mail at 4 o'clock in the afternoon. On Saturday, I got my mail at 5 o'clock. . . . I am on social security and my check is not made of rubber. When I pay my bills sometimes I have $4.00 left. Why don't they make the people who work for the government pay for the stamps? Make the President pay for his mail and not tax the people who are poor."

Mrs. "A," address unknown, writes the following letter: "I read on the front page of the *Guide* 'Kensington Pride Spreads.' You can print some of this. When this street cleaning pride began, I put a paper bag by my steps, in hope that people would use it. It helped. Even as far as children were concerned, we got them putting their goodie wrappings, cups and bottles in the bag. Guess what happened? A police car stopped in front of my house and when I asked if I could help him, he said he would have to give me a citation for having a bag of trash by my steps. I told him we were trying to teach the children to put their trash in it. He said that was nice, but I still had to take the bag inside. So how can you win? . . ."[13]

PR of "E." St. writes: "Last week, my trash was not picked up at the usual day or time. I saw three trucks parked a few blocks away from my house at 2:30 in the afternoon. These dedicated employees of the present corrupt city government were loitering about having themselves a holiday. My trash has always been taken away about 9:30 in the morning, but this time I had to wait until the next day. These guys are moaning and groaning about private contractors taking over their jobs, so why don't they do a little hustling and show us how a job can be done? They've been on easy street long enough with all the benefits they receive."

A letter from NG of "D" St. reads: "In answer to those who have written about the teachers' salary, I just have one little item to write. There are a group of teachers who travel together to their condos in Florida to spend the summer vacation. Why they go to a hot climate is beyond me, but they at least have been able to save from their miserable salaries and have a little of the good life. My heart bleeds for them!" I'm having a hard time controlling my tears and I also can't help but wonder why anybody would go to Florida in the summer, unless you live there.

SW of "E." St. writes: "I won't mention who won a bundle down the shore at one of the casinos, but she gets food stamps and welfare checks. You know who you are and you ought to be ashamed of yourself. My taxes go up on account of people like you. If you need the stamps or welfare, that's OK with me, but to go to the gambling places is beyond belief."

The general picture, through these and other passages, is strong and consistent. The government does not pay its own postage; police officers hassle decent, neighborly people when they should be ticketing speeding cars; the sanitation workers loiter about all day and are protected through powerful, highly paid union bosses; public school teachers with condos in Florida have the nerve to complain that their salaries are too low; and the welfare bureaucracy treats their clients to the easy life. The city government is corrupt, passing out patronage to some but leaving the river wards with insufficient services, except in election years. The complaint is clear: decent people who work hard and try their best are taken advantage of through high taxes that go for useless services and unfair advantages to others. Through stories about public employees and others who live on tax money, a general image of the public authority is constructed. The image is of an authority that is abusive, irrational, self-serving, and greedy. The claim that this authority works for the public good is held to be illegitimate.

The citizens of the river wards are represented, by their own letters and by Dan's exegesis, as both angry and insightful. They understand how the real world works, on a concrete level, and are not fooled or impressed by claims to authority. Neither are they fooled or impressed by people who assume a superior air, or think they are putting one over on the neighbors. The readers of the *Guide,* as represented in "by Dan," have a sharp eye for hypocrisy, for people who pretend to a lofty status. This hypocrisy engenders either amusement, as is often the case in tales of romance, or bitterness, which is expressed toward corrupt civil authorities. Both amusement and bitterness are savored as end points, with Dan and his readers in agreement that nothing essential will ever change. In either case, the readers of "by Dan" enjoy the satisfaction of feeling that they can see through the mechanisms of things and that other solid citizens in their neighborhood see things the same way.

Cancer, an important public issue in the river wards, is not discussed often in "by Dan." From time to time, smoking is discussed—the rights of smokers and nonsmokers in the workplace and in public is a favorite topic—and cancer risk is sometimes mentioned in this regard. But the link between cancer and pollution is rarely discussed. Following is one of the rare entries on this topic. The letter and Dan's reply took up an entire column. The writer focuses her complaints on a leading figure in a local protest group.

Dan: I am a 76-year-old widow, born and raised in the vicinity of the so-called Belway Company. I am in perfect health and have lived here most of my lifetime. . . . this area may be polluted by Belway or the Electric Company on the waterfront, but I doubt it can be that bad. I dare you to drive in front of this so-called Della Preszinski's house. In her front windows she has the most beautiful plants—geraniums—I've ever seen in Philadelphia. . . . Her plants are enormous, so the level around her house can't be too bad. Those toxins—if there are some—aren't killing her plants. She should have been in this locality 50–60 years ago. Melbourne opened valves every Monday, and the whole neighborhood reeked with a stench as though it was linseed oil, whatever it was. I have friends who live 30–40 miles from here in the country and in the mountains—no factories, no odors, no smoke, nothing—and still some have died from cancer. So I think the dame wants publicity. She has lived around here about one year; if that's so, what the heck does she know? Her neighbors were born in the houses (next door to hers) and they are OK." Well, this lady has some misinformation. For despite what she says, it has been proven that the Belway firm is releasing toxic fumes. . . . It is bad, despite what you think, and it's a shame that area residents have to be subjected to such pollution.

This echoes the common "by Dan" theme, as discussed above, of hostility between river wards people and outsiders who assume authoritative positions. A prominant thread in this passage involves reference to the antipollution activist as an outsider to the neighborhood.

As an element of discourse, this is held to invalidate her right to hold an opinion and discredit what she is saying. The use of "so-called" is interesting: the pose, if not the literal meaning, of this description implies that the terms of identity assumed by the protester are somehow false and insincere. Dan disagrees, calling it "a shame," a phrase which, in working-class Philadelphia, can carry a somewhat stronger moral disapproval than it does among some other subsets of speakers in the United States. As with the "by Dan" discourse on public employees, Dan's bottom line is anger about abuses of authority that are seen as inescapable: in the case at hand, pollution is imposed upon the people of the community, who "have to be subjected" to it.

The "by Dan" columns enjoin us to maintain our property, keep our behavior in line, and reject the intrusions of civic authority into neighborhood life. True river wards people, according to the voices in "by Dan," do not hold themselves apart from their neighbors. In fact, they derive great satisfaction and enjoyment from drawing on and living with expressions of community solidarity. In an important sense, "by Dan" represents a discourse on belonging and not belonging in the river wards. As we shall see, the issue of cancer and air pollution carries heavy reference to the same discourse.

The *Philadelphia Daily News,* the *Philadelphia Magazine,* and the *Guide* all carry distinct images of the river wards. In the *Daily News,* the river wards people are honest, struggling workers. In *Philadelphia Magazine,* they are disorganized families and social pathologies. In "by Dan," they want to know who asked anyone else's opinion. This voice sounds most like the internal voices of Tannerstown.

INSIDE AND OUTSIDE OF TANNERSTOWN

Some people describe Tannerstown as an open and friendly place, whereas others describe it as hostile and suspicious of strangers. I would not argue with either of these characterizations. But I feel most comfortable just saying that Tannerstown is a community with a good sense of its own borders. In this section, I will present Tannerstown voices on the topic of belonging and not belonging in the community.

Belonging

Through my work in Tannerstown, I met a woman whom I will call Dorothy, whose young daughter had developed a strange marking on her skin. Dorothy's immediate fear was cancer. I worked with Dorothy to identify the best local skin-cancer clinics. Of the institutions I recommended, she chose a clinic at one of the many teaching hospitals in Philadelphia. I helped her make the appointment for her daughter. During the next few months, I stayed in contact, calling or stopping by to find out how things were going. Dorothy was frightened as she saw her daughter through several appointments and tests and then elated at the eventual diagnosis of a nonmalignant condition. When she told me the good news, she made a point to add that she intended to speak positively to everyone she knew about the cancer education project for which I worked. With the urgency of a convert, she told me that she was going to "tell everyone" that "you really care." She added: "You're not just here—you know." Later, she came to an open house at our community clinic, and embraced me warmly in front of a crowd of her neighbors.

Dorothy had asked for practical assistance, and I had given it. But we had both experienced the transaction on another level. For both of us, the experience was, as anthropologists say, a breakdown—that is, a moment of rupture in the flow of normal, unexamined assumptions about social life. It came as a surprise to Dorothy that I was concerned enough to give her what was, considering my resources, a very simple kind of help. It came as a surprise to me that this surprised her. When she hugged me in the office, I was thrilled—not only because her daughter was healthy, but also because Dorothy had such warm feelings toward me. I felt that something in her perception of me, and of the cancer-education project, had changed. The sentence that began, "You're not just here—" implied that she had held a presumption that, as a representative of an organization based outside the community, my purpose was to take from or use Tannerstown in some way. Dorothy had presumed that my motives were not founded on person-to-person caring. My help with her daughter's case had turned this perception around.

The above story speaks to a strong sense of community boundaries. The "here" in "You're not just here—" is Tannerstown. People feel and frequently refer to the boundary between "us" and "them," between Tannerstown and the outside world. Another way this is expressed is through a strong sense of the physical borders of the neighborhood. This holds true for many river wards neighborhoods. It came into play early in the cancer-education campaign, when a project health educator organized the first meeting of the community advisory board. This board was made up of residents from several river wards neighborhoods. In one neighborhood, he told board members that the meeting was to be held in the next neighborhood. "But how would we get there?" they asked, bewildered. They were just blocks away, but it was the next neighborhood and therefore relatively unknown territory.

The physical borders of Tannerstown are, in fact, distinct. On one side, it is bordered by a complex of main roads. One woman I interviewed lived right on the other side of that border. When I called her to request an interview, she said, "I live on the other side of Maragona Avenue. I hope you don't mind coming over here." Her house turned out to be one block from Maragona. She is separated from Tannerstown by this very busy street and a walk, through underpasses, of about five blocks. She feels that she lives in the middle of nowhere and apologized to me for dragging me out of the neighborhood. She misses being in Tannerstown, she told me. She misses being able to walk to her mother's and her grandmother's with the kids.

Uh, in Tannerstown, I'd walk from one end of Tannerstown to the other every day, with my two kids, like to my mother's, I'd walk them to the park. I'd walk—and then I'd put all my children to bed and I'd go out myself, walk down again across Tannerstown to my girlfriend's, sit on the step at night and drink tea, walk home again, and in between I'm housecleaning and washing and what—and it was constantly. . . . I'm missing out on walking, I don't get out. Walking to the bar for a pack of cigarettes was so refreshing for me, that air.

In Tannerstown, residents say, everyone knows each other. People are used to living with the feeling that the people they know are all interconnected. If this is not so, it is felt as a disruption. Once, when I was talking with a Tannerstown woman about a nutrition education program with which she was helping, we were talking about other possible volunteers. She suggested one of her neighbors. How about Janie, she said? "You know Janie, don't you?" she asked. When I did not, she was stunned, momentarily speechless, not sure how to proceed.

Many community women spoke of this neighborhood familiarity:

I was born and raised here and my husband lived—well, he, too, more or less. He moved—he lived on this street when he was younger. Then he moved to [another river wards neighborhood], and then he moved back here, I think when he was in fourth or fifth grade. But he lived on Palmyra Street, right above Maragona Street. But he belonged to this parish. He was in my room in school. So it's one of those.

She describes her marriage as "one of those," as a familiar occurrence in neighborhood experience. In another passage from the same interview, she points to her children as central in building and maintaining her neighborhood networks:

It's a small community, you know. Everybody really knows each other or you know their faces from their kids. . . . They know your children, and the children know the parents, you know, even though you don't know— I'll go to Billy, "Who's he?" "Oh, he played basketball with me last year." You know, they see you picking up your child and then they get familiar with you.

Other Tannerstown women echo this:

It's really good here, you got the schools close by and stores. . . . It's a nice neighborhood, everybody knows everybody, and everybody watching out for everybody else. . . . In the summertime I can let the kids outside and soon as something goes wrong, one of my neighbors is telling me this and that's going on. . . . even let's say within this whole block, if something would happen, people are right there for you. Sometimes I think other neighborhoods, no. And then I know myself for a fact, like, the younger generation that are moving in. . . . I think that years ago, they were brought up here, and then for some reason, you know, "I want to get out of The Town" and then they move away and buy real expensive places and stuff like that. And they feel that they miss something. And they come back to The Town, you know. It's a nice little community. I mean, like I said, you know, there's, there are kids that are bad, and a little bit of drugs going on and stuff like that. But a lot of people here, I don't think tolerate it as much. You know what I mean? We do something about it. And if you say, "Hey, your kid was bad," sometimes they'll still listen and say, "Okay, I'll knock his block off."

For Tannerstown women, watching over each other's children is a key expression of communality.

I feel it's a safe place for the children to play. I don't like the idea of living on a main street, but I still have my yard. And I have a pool out there for us, so they really don't have much to worry about. I feel it's safer here— it's the truth—it's safer here than it is out in my mother's neighborhood— and my mother lives in a nice section. . . . Around here, everybody knows everybody. So if my kids went down two blocks over, I know somebody that's on that block and basically I know that they would keep an eye and when she sends her kids over here she knows I would keep an eye on them. In either direction, no matter where you go, I know somebody some- where in the neighborhood, and, you know, know that they're all right.

Of course, not everybody conforms to this communal vigilance over the children. But it is enough of a genuine community norm that people are subjected to criticism for removing themselves from the network:

You yell at not only your own but everybody else's, and you feel sorry for yelling at somebody else's kids because sometimes you get flak for that, you know? Like one time a neighbor—her child was—had chalk and was doing it on a house at the corner here, and I says, "Please don't do that." He goes, "It's okay," I said, "No, it's not." You know. So I called up the mother and she's a friend of mine, and I says, you know, "I told him not to do it, you know, in case he mentions it to you." And she goes, "That's all right. The rain will wash it off." But the rain doesn't wash it off. So I said from then on—it's—forget about this, you know?

Despite exceptions, most Tannerstown women seem to value the sense of shared neighborly authority over the children. The women quoted above, and others who spoke on the topic, made clear that they feel the need to keep a close eye on their children. But they say that it is easier to do this in Tannerstown. One afternoon, I was visiting in a Tannerstown home when school let out for the day. The woman I was visiting checked the time and opened her door. We stood on her porch, looking down the street at St. Joseph's parish school, watching her very young child walk two blocks home. There is a satisfaction to a life in which one can do this.

Through reference to these family issues, Tannerstown women point to the feeling of community they enjoy. In all my transcripts from interviews and focus groups (group interviews), I find only one passage in which a respondent, a woman from Tannerstown, speaks about community solidarity in abstract terms. (In this excerpt, as in others to follow, I have bracketed my own speech and identified it with my initials, MB):

I guess people around here just, you know, are just eager to make things work for themselves. But this has always been a community where people want things to happen for them. They just don't, uh, you know, let things go. They want to be part of things. They want to—you know, they just want everything to go smoothly and to be able to say, "Well, this is how it's going to work today, and tomorrow maybe we'll see whether we can do something a little differently." But, uh, if you have the will to do something, you're going to do it. If you don't, then nobody's going to change your mind about it. [MB: Are you talking about, like, um, kind of, taking charge of things by yourself type of thing? So there's a very clear independence?] Yeah. But it's an independence that works well with—you know, in a group, too. Because, you know, people can only—one person can only do so much and then they have to rely on, you know, other people to help them, too. So if they can work well alone, and with a group, then everything *can* work out.

At the time of this interview, I found this passage impossible to understand—my own initial misinterpretation is recorded in the above quotation—and I still find it to be difficult. But clearly, this woman is pointing to some of the themes addressed by the respondents quoted above: a willingness to pitch in and an optimism about working with one's neighbors. These themes form a positive image of the barrier between Tannerstown and the rest of the world.

Not Belonging

The opposite side of this coin is hostility toward outsiders, usually referred to as the ubiquitous "they." One thread of this, common to many in the United States, is a lament about economic loss and struggle. The following quotation from a focus-group participant is illustrative:

> The pay comes in, it's just not big enough. . . . Just getting the money to make the ends *meet* for what—for your everyday necessities. Not for luxury. To hell with luxury! I mean, hell! You know, we hope to get a vacation every year or every other year or whatever. It's just living day to day. And you just can't do it. They're, they're, they're—they're pushing us, *way* under. You just can't do it.

Because my record of Tannerstown talk is focused on attitudes toward cancer, the medical scientist emerges as the clearest personification of "they." Throughout the world, the scientist is a familiar figure in popular constructions of faceless authority and failure to see human meanings. We see this figure in popular literature and cinema, from Dr. Frankenstein to Dr. Strangelove. In Tannerstown, scientists and physicians who deal with cancer are the "they" who are most intimately owned by the community. For instance, "they" are often cast as responsible for science's failure to "find the cure."

> But I don't think they're—they can probably do a lot better. If we can send a man to the moon, how come we can't find the cure for cancer? There's so much research getting a man to the moon—what is the story for stopping us here?

Medical science is also incapable of straight answers regarding cancer and pollution in Tannerstown. The following quotation is from a long-time Tannerstowner, who now lives right outside the community borders:

When we first sent the kids down to St. Joe's, I was concerned because of all the factories around there. . . . I asked my doctor about it, and—the kids' doctor—and he said, "I really wouldn't worry about it." He said, "If you've got somebody in the house who's smoking," he says, "it's the same kind of toxic level as to have the kids down there *outside* with all that stuff from the factories." So since they had a smoker at home, I wasn't about to get myself all upset about the factories because, you know, clean up the home first before I start bugging *them*. You know, I was always—we grew up in the sixties—late sixties and seventies—and there was a whole thing about antipollution and all that and clean air. So it bothered me—well, it still bugs me that they have it, but, you know, where do you start? They tell you one thing, and it might be true and it might not be true.

In this passage, medical authority fails to deal in a satisfactory way with local concerns about cancer. Dissatisfaction with the responses of scientific medicine resonates with wider dissatisfactions about the "they" who pollute the neighborhood and then tell residents nothing useful or conclusive about cancer risks.

This passage shows clear resentment of "they" and defines "they" as not belonging to Tannerstown. But the issue of cancer and air pollution is not drawn in black and white. Tannerstowners are multivocal on the subject, both in the sense that there is variety in point of view and in the sense that within one person's statements a discourse of conflicting views can often be seen. The following quotation illustrates this.

I think it has a lot to do with the environment, myself . . . especially where we live here. You know that this is not—this is a nice area to live in but healthwise we have all these chemicals here and I don't care what anybody says, it's probably in—affected people. But, uh, I don't know—my son's family doctor told me to only live here for five years and move out. You know, he recommended that. But you can go anywhere and you're going to hit it. I don't care what anybody says.

Twice, this Tannerstown woman shifts her stance. With the words "But, uh, I don't know—," she hints that she might debate what she has said up until that point. At the end of that phrase, she breaks off, quoting her son's doctor to support her original point. But then she debates herself with "But you can go anywhere." The final phrase, "I don't care what anybody says," shows her definition of this topic as a hotly debated one.

One strong community voice does assert that only outsiders tie Tannerstown's high cancer rates to local pollution. In the following quotation, one sees very clearly the interweaving of the issue of belonging and not belonging in Tannerstown with that of attitudes toward the area's high cancer rates. At the beginning of this interview excerpt, I had left the subject of cancer behind several questions ago. But when I asked this woman about her length of residence in Tannerstown, she jumped right back to it.

[MB: Has your family lived in Tannerstown for a long time?] Yeah, that too, cancer from Tannerstown, yeah, but I—like, people tell me that. Like, with the Drug Mart opening up down the street here, there's people coming from different areas, like my manager and stuff like that. So I said, like, they, you know, they would say something about, you know, "This was on TV about being cancerous." And I'd say, "Well, there's people have been living here for eighty years and they're still here and they might be healthier than you." You know, so, it's hard, you know. So, like, right now, I don't think—it scares me, but it doesn't. Because there's so much of it. So, you know. But I know Tannerstown, it's been on TV, you know. Announced, you know, and whatsoever. But I'm here and I love it here, you know, and it's—to me, you can get it anywhere and anytime, the way there's so much of it, and different kinds. So maybe with the chemicals, it might push it a little bit faster, but you're gonna get it or you're not gonna get it.

In this passage, the speaker defines an outside voice and an inside voice in the debate about Tannerstown's cancer rates. The voice that describes Tannerstown as being, essentially and centrally, a "cancer zone" is defined as external, that of "people coming from different areas." Her own voice, which she defines as native, says, "I'm here and I love it here," and goes on to question the extent to which living in Tannerstown determines one's risk of acquiring cancer. She is clear as to her position, but her discourse reveals that the debate between the two voices is a difficult one.

This is dramatically illustrated by an exchange among participants in one of the focus groups early in the project. This exchange, quoted below at some length, is among several participants (P1–P6) and the facilitator (F), one of the project health educators. In this passage, the participants discuss an incident in the early 1980s in which a major industrial accident at one of the nearby chemical plants caused Tannerstown to be temporarily cordoned off. The passage shows us multiple points of view about the accident and a simultaneous discourse about which of these points of view belong or do not belong in Tannerstown.

This material is transcribed in more detail than other material presented in this book: opening brackets are used to indicate interruptions and simultaneous beginnings; interruptions are indicated directly below the precise word on which they begin; "PX" is used where the identity of the speaker is not clear; and "xxxxxx" indicates sections of inaudible speech.

1	P1	And I think the majority of people around
2		here feel that way.
3	F	M-hm.
4	P1	You know, because most of the people that
5		live in Tannerstown, I mean, we've read in
6		the paper and all that we're a high-cancer-
7		risk area. Most people that live in
8		Tannerstown, you would have a hard time
9		convincing about that.
10	F	That—that—
11	P1	That this is a high cancer area.
12	F	Really?
13	P1	[Because we have
14	P2	[I think it's the newer people—
15	P1	a *lot,* of older people, I mean *old* people,
16	P2	Old, *old* people [*Laughter*]
17	P1	I'm talking in their nineties
18	F	M-hm.
19	P1	that are still walking around and
20		healthier than maybe you or I
21	PX	[And lived here all their life
22	P1	And lived here all their life.

23	F	M-hm.
24	P1	So it's going to be hard to convince anyone
25		that this is a high—even though we have
26		General Chemical, we have Wanser and Deetz,
27		you know
28	F	[M-hm.
29	P1	and at one time we had Consolidated Coke. And
30		then we now have—we have the—what is that
31		thing that burns these stinky things outside?
32	P3	[O-o-o-h
33	P2	[The water pollution (xxxxxx)
34	PX	[*That* thing. That—
35		that's worse than
36	PX	[O-o-h, o-o-h, yeah.
37	F	[What is that? The city goes in—
38	P1	[Right on Maxwell Street.
39	P2	[The city doesn't, uh, smellin' it, you know?
40	F	Today I did, I didn't the other time, yeah
41	P2	[The city's the
42		worst offender, I feel
43	P1	[That's the city.
44	P2	I really do.
45	P1	[Right.
46	F	M-hm.
47	P1	Because it'sa, it's the different city
48		things, that cause the smell in here, and
49		people will know
50	PX	[It's enough to make you sick
51	P1	as soon as they enter, "Oo, what is that
52		smell?"
53	F	M-hm.
54	P1	You know, and living here all our lives,
55		don't *smell* it.
56	F	M-hm.
57	P1	And people say, "Oh, how could you live in
58		this stinky part of, eeyoo
59	P4	[My husband said that when he
60		dated me. You know? [*Laughter*] "Can't even
61		pick you up and get you out of this place I—
62	P1	[Never bothered
63		me. But I think the majority
64		would have a hard time convincing *anybody*,

65		that this was a high cancer area.
66	P3	Unless they didn't grow up here.
67	P1	[Unless they didn't—
68	PX	[Yeah.
69	PX	We've got people that moved in here that'll
70		complain like crazy. But I mean, they,
71		they've never *lived* here. I mean—
72	P1	I figure, if they hated it that bad, why'd ya
73		move here? [*Laughter*]
74	P1	And I feel terrible, I get up—
75	F	You *do* say that to them!?
76	P1	[I *do* get up to them. And what
77		frightens people more is not the cancer, I
78		don't think, as the risk of one of these
79		plants blowing up. Going to kingdom come.
80	P2	Right.
81	P1	Because we had—just this explosion last year
82		or a year or so ago. And a family *actually*
83		*sold* their home and *moved* out of Tannerstown
84		because *that* place blew *up.*
85	P2	And it blows up every year.
86	P1	And it blows up every Easter. [*Laughter.*
87		*Below: tone of amused enjoyment.*]
88	PX	Right.
89	PX	Every other Easter.
90	PX	It's about every Easter, though,
91		it's the truth.
92	P1	[It's always Easter week and it always blows
93		up, and it's always (xxxxxx), so, you know
94		[*End tone of amused enjoyment.*]
95	F	And that doesn't bother you.
96	P1	No.
97	F	You're just used to it cause you know—
98	P	I think there's safe—
99	PX	[xxxxxx]
100	P1	You know they got the safe precautions.
101		[*Laughter, relaxed tone*]
102		[We're getting out of—(xxxxxx)
103	P5	[(xxxxxx) first time I
104		experienced that, and I'll tell you I was
105		frightened.

106	P3	I was scared, too.
107	P1	It took me an hour and a half to get ba—I
108		wasn't in Tannerstown, it took me an hour and
109		a half to get back *into* Tannerstown and
110		*two* hours
111	P5	(xxxxxx), I wanted to get *out*—
112	P1	two-*two* hours, to get from Oaten Lane to
113		Northeast Avenue.
114	P5	Uh-huh.
115	P3	[Oh, my God.
116	P1	The—the police said won't—I said, "I have
117		family here." They said, "Well, that's too
118		bad, you park your car here and you can *walk*
119	P2	[And *walk,* that day,
120		yeah, you had to walk
121	P1	[into Tannerstown. And I said, well, that
122		doesn't make any *sense,* I'm gonna *walk* into
123		Tannerstown, I have a better chance if I'm
124		*ridin*'!
125	P3	That's right.
126	F	M-hm
127	P1	[Right. That's one of their main concerns,
128		more—more so than having—this being a high
129		cancer area.
130	F	M-hm. M-hm.
131	P1	Cause I have known people to move *out* because
132		they thought the place was gonna blow up.
133	P3	[M-hm.
134	P6	[Everything got so dark and the
135		windows just shook—Oh, it was terrible! And
136		the kids were getting out of school, like,
137		then—
138	P3	The kids.
139	P1	[Yeah, that was the scariest part. Cause I
140	P6	[(xxxxxx) and the sidewalks were all—
141	P1	walked down—out of here with
142		mine—
143	P3	My kids were screaming bloody murder running
144		down the street.
145	P1	Yeah.
146	F	Oh, it must have been frightening for them.

147	P3	[Yes.
148	P6	Well, my grandfather—gettin' out,
149	P1	[Well, we're not too far away from
150	P6	you know—
151	P1	[you—here, you would hear the—the—the
152		repercussion of the, of the explosion. Right.
153	P6	Yeah.
154	P1	[See now when I was a *child,*
155		growing up, I lived across the
156		*street* from the General plant.
157	P3	[So you had your windows blown out how many
158		times?
159	P1	[So my windows blew
160		out.
161	P3	Yeah.
162	P1	See, so whena—when that happens, (xxxxxx)
163	P2	[When you get the
164		repercussions it's nothin'! [*Laughter*]
165	PX	[No.
166	P1	We're comin' over [Interstate] 95 and—
167		somebody—'O-oh, well, General Chemical must
168		of blown up.' Didn't bother *me.* Cause I was
169		so *used* to it from,
170	P3	Yeah.
171	P1	from a child,
172	F	Mm.
173	PX	[Um-hm.
174	P1	knowing that this thing is gonna blow every
175		Easter. . . . That's why us oldies don't have
176		the fear here that the new ones coming in,
177		when you see them on TV, cause my brother-in-
178		law could pinpoint 'em cause they're at his
179		door every, every *day.*
180	F	M-hm.
181	P1	You know, these are people that *didn't* live
182		here, so naturally, they're gonna go to *them—*
183		"What do you think of it?" "Well, it's
184		*rotten,* it's no *good,* get *rid* of 'em" and all
185		that. We grew *up* with all this.
186	P2	I love the ones that demonstrate. They have
187		nothing better to do just to go by—by a
188		company and demonstrate. The—*I* never seen

189		these people in my *life*,
190	PX	Mm.
191	P2	and I've lived here all my *life*.
192	P1	Right.
193	P2	*Where'd they come from?* They must have
194		imported them from another—place to cause
195		trouble.

In this dialogue, we hear a voice, most clearly represented by P1, P2, and P3, that claims to be the sole legitimate voice of Tannerstown. At lines 1–9, P1 represents herself as speaking for "most of the people that live in Tannerstown." As other respondents say, it is "the newer people" (line 14) who "complain like crazy" (line 70). But "they've never *lived* here" (line 71). This is echoed by P1 at lines 181–82, and by P2 at lines 188–91: "*I* never seen these people in my *life*, and I've lived here all my *life*." The tone of P2's emphatic "*Where'd they come from?*" (line 193) is the most dramatically emotional statement in the excerpt: it sounds based in righteous anger. The subjects of this anger, imported by "they" (lines 193–94), are the type of people who move out when General Chemical blows up. According to P1 and others, the true Tannerstowner knows that the plant "blows up every Easter" (lines 86–100). Like Easter, this is part of the life of the year, familiar ground for Tannerstowners, memories to laugh and shake your head about. At least, this is what the voice represented by P1 and others would have the facilitator believe.

At line 103, P5 voices her view of the explosion. To her, it was extraordinary and frightening. She introduces this statement in the midst of a hubbub of voices and laughter, which masks the moment at which she begins the statement. Neither she nor P6 (see line 134) challenge P1 in direct terms. Neither do they get very far with their statements. P5 begins at line 103 with enough sincerity to provoke a sympathetic remark from P3. P1, however, insists on regaining and keeping the floor for her position, fighting off challenges at line 111 and at line 119. She keeps the floor until the dialogue calms and slows at line 130. At line 134, P6 offers her challenge, which P1 silences by line 153, at which P6 is reduced to a weak "Yeah." In general, P1 is a very dominating voice, and interrupts other participants and the facilitator readily. But she is particularly eager to do so when she is confronted by a challenge on this topic.

This focus-group dynamic mirrors one that I have seen in many community settings. Divergent voices are present, and a debate ensues, sometimes more directly than shown here, about the role of local industry in cancer causation. In fact, as material presented later will show, the voice represented by P1 is not the only legitimate voice in Tannerstown. But her claim to sole legitimacy loads the debate on cancer and industry with other meanings and intertwines it with other debates. The passage quoted above is polysemous: it is about cancer risk, unwelcome intrusions, loyalties to local institutions, shared memories, and infuriating outsiders. Most central to my point, it is about belonging and not belonging in Tannerstown.

The river wards have a high-profile image in Philadelphia. Whether people know the area at first hand or just by reputation, it is an area about which people hold images and opinions. Many people point freely to the river wards when they talk about urban decay, white racism, ignorance, and poverty. To their eyes, it makes sense that the river wards are a cancer hot spot: they see it as something that the residents of the area have created, just as they have created their other problems.

Within the river wards, there is a diversity of opinion about the area's high cancer rates. Some agree that lifestyle is involved; some deny it and blame the cancer on pollution; some deny that pollution is at fault either, and they even doubt that cancer rates in the area really are high. But whatever their view, most river wards people deeply resent the criticism of outsiders and the tendency of outsiders to think of the river wards as a "cancer zone."

Central voices in the river wards identify the authority of science as one source of such outside criticism. This characterization is particularly strong in Tannerstown, where the high cancer risk, which most people believe to be real, is the backdrop against which issues regarding power and pollution are thrown into high relief. In Tannerstown it has become a master issue to which other issues are linked and through which discourse on other issues may be expressed. Talking about cancer is often a code for talking about other things.

PROJECT CAN-DO $\boxed{3}$

April has been proclaimed "Cancer Control Month" in the United States.
While the rest of the country is *talking* about taking control of cancer,
Project CAN-DO is helping people to *do* something about it.
The Guide, May 1, 1987

You can't do anything about it.
Tannerstown resident

Project CAN-DO was a five-year cancer-education campaign, under-
taken from 1983 to 1988 in seven river wards neighborhoods in Philadelphia. The project was directed by cancer-control researchers from
the Fox Chase Cancer Center and funded by the National Cancer
Institute. Project staffing was modest: a director (the principal investigator), two health educators, two data analysts, and one administrative assistant. Other resources were also limited; the project staff was
responsible for virtually all design of new print and audiovisual materials, as well as for program delivery and data collection and analysis.
Within these limitations, project researchers had proposed to serve a
population of about 100,000.

In previous descriptions of Project CAN-DO, the seven neighborhoods that project leaders originally planned to serve are described as
"the Project CAN-DO community." As explained below, three of the
seven neighborhoods were later singled out to receive more intensive
attention. Tannerstown was one of those three.

Project CAN-DO was modeled after several successful community-
based projects that had focused on the prevention of heart disease (Farquhar et al. 1977; Puska et al. 1976). It was to serve as a test of whether
these community-based models would be effective in cancer-control

work. Project CAN-DO planners started with the assumption that the experiences of the researchers on heart disease would serve as a general guide for what they might expect to face in the field. Nothing could have been further from the truth.

The five-year plan for Project CAN-DO called for a baseline survey in the first year to measure existing cancer-related knowledge, attitudes, and practices in the study community. The following three years were to include media campaigns, educational programs, and provision of cancer-testing services at a community site. In the fourth project year, the survey was to be repeated. In the fifth and final year, project researchers would conduct an analysis, comparing data from the two surveys to test for any changes in knowledge, attitudes, and practices.

As planned, the project began with the baseline survey. This survey, distributed by mail, included a series of questions on knowledge of and attitudes and practices toward cancer. As a control condition, a set of nearly identical questions on heart disease was included. The return rate was 23 percent—low, but not unexpectedly so for a mail survey of a general population on a sensitive topic. From a comparison of survey and census data, it appeared that survey respondents had more formal education and a somewhat higher income than average for the river wards. Compared with respondents to other surveys of the general population of the United States, respondents to this survey seemed very knowledgeable about cancer, and a very high proportion of them reported knowing someone with cancer (Amsel et al. 1986).

The researchers were struck, however, by another aspect of the results. Among the survey respondents, attitudes toward cancer were significantly and consistently more negative than attitudes toward heart disease. Respondents indicated that they were frightened of and pessimistic about cancer. This raised questions about whether the heart disease projects would serve as a good model for cancer control in the river wards. After consultation with the project's community advisory board, planners of the project decided to do more intensive work in a smaller geographical area. Three neighborhoods, as mentioned above, were chosen for this more intensive effort. The project director was eager to find ways to devote even more project time and effort to understanding community beliefs about cancer.

The project was begun, and the name "Project CAN-DO" was chosen. This name reflected the official philosophy of the project: that with regard to cancer prevention, we should focus on factors within our personal control—on the things that we all "can do" to reduce our risk of cancer. In other words, Tannerstowners were advised to adopt lifestyle changes—to quit smoking, change their diet, and go for regular cancer screening—to adapt to life in the "cancer zone."

HEALTH EDUCATION PRACTICE

My own involvement with Project CAN-DO began one year after the program had begun. By this time, it was clear that community resistance to project messages was profound. The project director hired me partly because of my background in anthropology: she hoped that I could unravel some of the threads of the community's resistance. As indicated above, she saw this resistance as a critical research focus in its own right. In this, she was daring and creative beyond the bounds of the external strictures on her. My duties, as she assigned them, were to develop and deliver educational programs and to conduct an ethnographic substudy on community attitudes toward cancer.

These two sets of duties defined two different roles for me in the community. On one hand, I was a health educator and as such spent countless hours in community schools, attended various community events, and sat in on meetings of the Home and School Association (parent-teacher association), senior citizens' groups, community leaders, and our project advisory board. On the other hand, I was an anthropologist and spent informal time with people—at first interviewing them and then, later, visiting with community friends. In both roles, I heard a lot of talk about cancer.

My time to be an anthropologist was always very limited. The project's schedule for program design and implementation was fierce, and I came in at a busy time. Doing ethnography faded into the background as I threw myself into doing educational presentations at schools and community group meetings. This work offered me an odd window into the community—one clouded a bit by the community's neighborly hospitality but still clear enough to transmit some pretty strong objections to the lessons I was teaching.

An Evening's Work

The reader is asked to imagine a large meeting hall in the basement of a Catholic church. The floor is linoleum and the walls yellowish green, with grates over high, small windows. There are fifty or sixty people there, mostly women, for the monthly meeting of the Home and School Association. The people all know each other and laugh and joke about recent shared events. Seven or eight women are crammed into a kitchen designed for two, all busily helping to get the coffee on. Ten trays of donuts, cakes, and cookies await the end of the formal meeting. Several sisters from the teaching order are present, including the principal of the church school, who is accorded great respect. The pastor is also present and delights his parishioners with an energetic display of informality and folksy humor.

The Project CAN-DO team, consisting of myself and a colleague, arrives, carrying a box of pamphlets, a box of survey forms, Project CAN-DO pencils for the respondents to use and then keep, a gift-wrapped box with a prize to raffle off, a tray of slides, a fifty-foot-long orange extension cord, a wall plug adaptor, a slide and tape projector, and assorted demonstration paraphernalia. We find the president of the Home and School Association, who beams at me. "Oh," she says, "you're the cancer lady. Well, let's get you settled in!" There is some excitement involved in finding us a place to put all our things. Finally, the projector is set up on an old piano bench, propped up by a stack of books. The slides will be shown on a wall, lending a yellowish green tint to the entire production.

The meeting begins. Business is first, consisting of the treasurer's report on the recent car wash, which earned enough to buy a computer for the eighth graders. A woman from a nearby parish is introduced. Carefully coiffed and tailored, she is there to recruit women to clean downtown office buildings at night. The pastor then addresses the audience, gently urging them to support the upcoming holy communion celebration. The meeting has lasted about twenty minutes, and the mood is friendly. The association president then announces "the lady from the CAN-DO," who will address the audience on the high-fiber, low-fat diet.

I talk a few minutes, guide the audience through a written questionnaire, and present a slide show. After the slides, I ask if there are any questions. I look out at a sea of faces, all of which look silently back. Some hard work on my part brings out a few comments, mostly brief testimonials from women who already use chicken hot dogs, who have already switched to skim milk, who have done this and more because it is good for their hearts. After these few comments, the silence returns. I bring out a rubber model of five pounds of body fat, which engenders much joking and laughing. I raffle off a hot-air popcorn maker, to the delight of all concerned. I then ask if there are any more questions, and the silence immediately returns. I smile, thank the audience, and the meeting adjourns to coffee and cake.

Over coffee and cake, subterranean matters surface. "My sister had cancer," confides one woman, "and the doctors couldn't do nothing for her." "I have a neighbor who eats the old food, and she is ninety-three years old, would you like to meet her?" says another, with a joking but pointed spirit. "You mean, your husband will eat that stuff? Mine won't," says a third. "You'll never convince most of these people," says the last, "they like their kielbasa too much. Come by the next church dinner for some really good eating," she adds.

Then, the social climax: I am offered a piece of cake. The offerer, and a goodly number of onlookers, can barely restrain their hilarity. Time stops. Then I accept the cake. There is a burst of teasing and laughter, the conversation becomes easier, and then the moment passes. We eat, pack our equipment, and leave.

The general mood of these meetings is friendly, but the health-education messages are met with silence. According to one of the women I interviewed, there is social pressure not to speak:

[MB: The nutrition show that we just showed at Saint Sebastian's, um— afterwards there weren't any questions. So it's hard for me—and that was the first time we had shown it. It's hard for me to think, well, what are people thinking?] . . . I did have questions and came to you afterwards. Cause some of the people, not that I care, I really don't care what they think of me. But I heard a few, like, "well, now we can go." So I didn't want to hold back anyone. That's why I came up to you. Afterwards.

"I really don't care what they think of me," she says. This phrase marks a well-worn point of contention in the river wards communities: accepting or rejecting the advice of outside scientific experts.

Specific Moments, Humiliating and Otherwise

Being a health educator for Project CAN-DO was hard work. Community health education in general tends to be hard work. Along with our colleagues from other projects, the Project CAN-DO field staff developed comedic traditions that helped us all deal with the stress we felt.

One such tradition was entitled "Humiliating Moments in Health Education."[1] This was the title of a session that we were always fictitiously planning to present at the annual meeting of the American Public Health Association. At regular lunches and meetings, Fox Chase researchers and health educators swapped stories that we could write papers about for such a session. Those of us who worked on Project CAN-DO contributed our fair share of stories.

One "humiliating moment" was experienced early on by the entire Project CAN-DO staff while passing out copies of the pilot version of the baseline survey after Sunday morning services at a Tannerstown church. The parish priest was supportive of this activity and had promised to announce it from the pulpit. Unfortunately, he chose that day's sermon to lecture against the evils of a bizarre religious sect, members of which had in recent weeks been handing out leaflets to local churchgoers after Sunday morning services. Imagine the shock of the Project CAN-DO staff when scores of churchgoers angrily shunned their offered surveys, mistaking project staff for sect members. One devout parishioner was especially enthusiastic: he spit on the CAN-DO staffers.

Then there was the lottery, designed to increase the return rate for the baseline survey. One lucky survey respondent was to win $300. The winning number belonged to a woman whose survey had been addressed simply to the occupant of her address. A project staffer called on her home, to tell her she had won. But the lucky winner refused to give her name, stating that she wanted to maintain her anonymity and wanting to know who we were, anyway. This made it impossible to write her a check for her winnings. Finally, her husband persuaded her to give her name—he wanted the money. But our project staffer returned feeling humiliated, when he had least expected to be met with rejection.

Another story involves a health educator who joined the project after some initial work had already been done. He remembered his very first presentation to a community group:

I spoke with the Dell Home and School Association about the fact that, ah—try to negate some of the perceptions of cancer—we call them the myths or the misconceptions about cancer, that it's everywhere, that there's nothing people can do to prevent it, and I was trying to let them know that there *were* things, you know, and, um, one very indignant woman interrupted me, interrupted the whole proceeding—heavy Polish accent, but a young woman, no more than twenty-five years old—how dare I come into her community and tell them they don't know how to live their lives, that it's their own fault, and, ah—people were too polite to let her continue, but I think she was speaking for a large proportion of the population.

Some time later, a project health educator wrote a series of articles for the community newspapers. In each article, he included our phone number and urged readers with questions to call. There were not many calls, but one staff member got a call from a reader who asked point by point if everything in the article was true: if you don't smoke, if you eat right, if you follow all these other recommendations and do all these things that are within your control, is it true that you lower your risk of cancer? Yes, our staff member said, that was right. Then why, the caller retorted, did the dog get cancer? My neighbor's dog just died of cancer. Why did the dog die of cancer? The dog didn't smoke, the dog didn't eat an improper diet, the dog didn't lay out in the sun. So why? The staff member who received that call was demoralized for some time after.

Later in the project, I ran a recipe contest as part of a campaign to encourage high-fiber, low-fat diets. Students in the schools we visited took the contest entries home to be filled out by a parent. "Send us a recipe for a traditional dish or an old family favorite!" the entry blank read. "Our nutritionist may suggest small changes in the winning recipes, which we will note when we print the winners." The nutritionist's role was to suggest changes whereby traditional favorites could be made higher in fiber or lower in fat. At least one contestant from the Tannerstown Polish parish took this as a challenge. He sent in the following recipe:

NAME OF DISH: The Polish Traditional Feast

INGREDIENTS: 5 lbs. fresh kielbasa (not smoked)
                     5 lbs. sauerkraut

INSTRUCTIONS: Place kielbasa in a large pot and cover with water. Bring to a boil and simmer for 45 min. and add sauerkraut. Continue to simmer for 30 minutes. Serve with horseradish or mustard.

SERVES: 14 people or 7 Polish people

Needless to say, the nutritionist was stumped.

We referred to these events, and many others like them, as "humiliating moments," and encouraged each other to read them as an isolated string of stories, like a stand-up comic routine. This tradition helped us to deal with our discouragement. The knowledge that community rejection of our messages was real engendered more than discouragement, however. We also admired the community's spirit and laughed at the humor of the people who were rejecting our messages. We ended up with a strong affiliation with the community.

Several years after the project ended, in an interview with the former director, I asked about her bottom-line perceptions of the Project CAN-DO community. She spoke of the issue of belonging—of discouragements but also of moments of connection. She remembered the kick-off meeting for the three-year community-based project:

It was funny—the kick-off meeting, um—I remember the dress—I bought a dress purposefully for the kick-off meeting, and it was a red dress with [a] white design—pattern on it. . . . I was very nervous about [the meeting] . . . . It was in a big hall and, ah, I talked about the project. I was very nervous about it, I didn't want to make it sound cold, or we were imposing on the community, because I wanted the community to really own it, um, but not sure how to do that, and I remember opening up for questions, and, no questions at first. And then, who raises their hand to ask a question but Rachel, eight-year-old Rachel, front row, and she wanted to know about why people—something about lung cancer—why people continued to smoke if they knew that [*Laughs*], "Mommy," and I said, "Uh, that's my daughter." And it wasn't a set-up. And it sort of broke the ice. And, um, afterwards when I came off the stage, and we sort of broke up, people came up to me and, um—one woman in particular came up to me and she said, "I have skin cancer on my arms," and I said, " 'Oh!" and she said, "I've never told anybody—I mean I've been to the doctor but nobody knows about it and I always wear long sleeve shirts." But she came up to me to do that, and that really made the—that's—I mean, that was such a warm—made me feel like I was part of the community.

A new dress and a big hall—the project director felt a sense of insecurity about being accepted in the community. Yet, small gestures speak loudly when one yearns for acceptance, and, fearing public rejection, she is grateful for any sign of support. Years later, her basic feeling toward the community is one of affiliation of sorts. This affiliation is loaded with peril, however. It does not square with the ideal of scientific detachment. The project director goes on:

I just found the people to be so, um—maybe it's because there is this distance between the people in that community and people outside that community. And the fact that I felt like they were willing to accept me was a major thing, and I really appreciated it. Maybe that's what it was. So they became people to me and I didn't maintain the detachment that I wanted to. But, um, I think in the long run it was better for the project that we didn't.

As so often happens, working in a community setting challenged the models and plans that researchers had constructed. Learned professional roles were unraveling. The community's voice was unsettling. The community had its own strong point of view, and it demanded engagement. Project CAN-DO field staff became inclined to listen. We were, however, confined by the "CAN-DO" philosophy—the philosophy that had been proposed to and funded by the National Cancer Institute, the philosophy that was internally approved at Fox Chase, the philosophy that was informed by approved theory in social psychology and that accorded with professional health-education practice. It was difficult to create a way out of this confinement, which shaped the form and determined the content of what we said to people. It was hard to get around it.

The Seven Misconceptions

The basic epistemology of Project CAN-DO—the project staff's received way of knowing and way of thinking about its goals and its study community—may be illustrated by looking at a list called the "seven misconceptions" about cancer. This list of seven statements of belief was developed from a literal reading of four early Project CAN-DO focus groups. These seven beliefs were identified as being common among community residents and as working against acceptance of Project CAN-DO messages. The seven misconceptions are as follows:

1. There is nothing you can do to prevent cancer.
2. There is cancer hidden in everybody. It is a matter of time until it becomes activated.
3. Cancer can be triggered by a bruise or blow to the body (often, but not exclusively, said about breast cancer).
4. Cancer is inherited. You can be born with it in your body.
5. Surgery can cause cancer to spread.
6. Cancer treatment is worse than the disease itself.
7. Cancer is a death sentence.

When these seven statements were first compiled as a list, they were referred to as the seven "myths" about cancer. A key staff member insisted that this be changed to the seven "misconceptions." This staffer was uncomfortable with "myths": "It made people sound less—I don't know what the word for it is—[*Pause*]—less—[*Pause*]—literate. Where 'misconceptions' was, the idea's right, but you're off base, or you've got the idea turned around. But 'myth' made it sound like it was make-believe."

This shift reflects a sense of discomfort that came to the fore through work in the community. In an essential sense, Project CAN-DO defined the community in terms of what was wrong, what needed changing. The list of seven statements about cancer, whether they are called myths or misconceptions, codified that. Confronting people from within this conceptual framework was extremely difficult, if you were at all inclined, as the staffer goes on to say, to "feel like they were real people and not just that community that didn't know anything. . . . [Calling them misconceptions] made it a bit more comfortable on my part. I think I told you the story about the woman who got up and said, 'How dare you'? That type of thing was always in the back of my mind."

Indeed, it was uncomfortable to confront the community with a list that purported to be a list of its own misconceptions. But professional health-education practice required that the community be viewed as in need of fixing and that the project's goal be to fix it. The right way to start, according to professional dictates, was with an educational diagnosis: that is, with a determination of the nature of the community's need to be taught. The list of seven "misconceptions" provided Project CAN-DO with a concrete educational goal: refute the seven misconceptions (see Workman et al. 1988).

If we consider these seven statements one by one, it becomes clear that they are not exactly either myths or misconceptions. The first statement is true enough, depending on how you read it: there is nothing you can do that will absolutely guarantee that you will not get cancer. The second statement reflects an understandable interpretation of scientific findings, widely reported in the popular press, that trace how some cancers develop through a series of precancerous events. With regard to the third statement, there is some evidence that physical trauma, especially if it is associated with chronic inflammation, may sometimes enhance the growth or spread of a preexisting cancer (see review in Weiss 1990). The fourth statement can also be read as loosely based on scientific fact: only a few rare forms of cancer are actually inherited, but the inheritance of risk factors is evidently very important in a number of common types of cancer (for instance, skin, breast, and colorectal). In addition, some babies are born with tumors. There is also a basis for the fifth statement. As discussed earlier, cancer surgery does cause showers of cancer cells to be released into the bloodstream, and some research does suggest, albeit indirectly, that this may pose special risks for residents of areas with high ambient air pollution (Richters 1988). The sixth statement—that cancer treatment is worse than the disease itself—is a subjective assessment, and it is certainly voiced often by cancer patients and those who are close to them. The seventh statement—that cancer is a death sentence—is hyperbole, but considering that the five-year relative survival rate for all cancer patients presently stands at about 50 percent, it is not an irrational statement, either.

On the whole, then, the seven misconceptions are no more disconnected to accurate cancer knowledge than are the denials of them that were promoted through Project CAN-DO. But it was predetermined that the community was to be defined as possessing a problem, and the seven misconceptions painted a familiar picture: working-class fatalism. This process of codification, of "educational diagnosis," was the professionally correct way to proceed. It replaced any more subtle, nonliteral assessment of the genesis or social meaning of each of the seven statements, or of messages lying behind the list as a whole.

In the Middle

Scientific medicine is a jealous discipline. It dictates, as a central article of faith, that the only valid road to health is paved with its own recommendations. Health behaviors and beliefs are beyond moral criticism only if they remain on this road. Otherwise, they are problematic and are cast as abnormalities through the process of medicalization (Illich 1977; Zola 1972). Scheper-Hughes and Lock summarize this concept as one that describes how:

[n]egative social sentiments . . . can be recast as individual pathologies and "symptoms" rather than as socially significant "signs." This funneling of diffuse but real complaints into the idiom of sickness has led to the problem of "medicalization" and to the overproduction of illness in contemporary advanced industrial societies. In this process the role of doctors, social workers, psychiatrists, and criminologists as agents of social consensus is pivotal . . . . the medical gaze is, then, a controlling gaze, through which active (although furtive) forms of protest are transformed into passive acts of "breakdown." (Scheper-Hughes and Lock 1987:27)

Adjunct health professionals, health educators among them, are often concerned to gain legitimacy in the eyes of physicians. This means affiliating themselves with the paradigm of scientific medicine. One way to do this is to adopt a clinical gaze, and to assume the role of diagnostician while looking at social life. Through a clinical gaze, the health educator may see those who do not follow scientific medical advice as being essentially sick. In the case described here, the diagnosis is fatalism. This fatalism is seen as situated within the individual, like an ear infection or a swollen appendix, or within a community or other social grouping as a whole. Like gaze and diagnosis, treatment is aggressive. The magic bullet is the health-education message, delivered to the target population through an appropriate strategy, preferably at a teachable moment. In this military language, describing health education's front in the war against cancer, we see the diffusion and elaboration of one of scientific medicine's fundamental metaphors (see Martin 1988).

Medicalization is implicit in the concept of working-class fatalism, and it is not officially recognized by either physicians or health educators. The process nonetheless functions to recast resistance to health-promotion efforts as a diagnosable pathology. Thus, the worldview of medical science is reproduced in a new setting. This may serve to make health-promotion efforts to "combat fatalism" seem more legitimate to the physicians on whose acceptance health-education researchers depend.

This medicalization has at least four consequences. First, it blocks the health educator's view. Along with the clinical gaze comes a pair of blinders. If fatalism is a disease, there is no need to look further at an indigenous etiology that is merely a symptom of this disease. Such an etiology may be dismissed as irrational, and the discourse between project and community may be understood only in narrow, adversarial terms.

Second, it obviates the need to develop a critical understanding of the beliefs held by health educators. Without such understanding, health educators have no razor, independent of that of medical science, with which to separate legitimate practice from delusion. In the case at hand, the health educator's selling of optimism about the curability of cancer must be examined as problematic, as a matter of ideology.

Third, it generates a conceptual schema that allows health professionals to ignore the insights and views of entire communities. With a diagnosis of fatalism, health educators provide clinicians, epidemiologists, and laboratory researchers a vocabulary with which to explain and dismiss the fears of working-class persons and groups. Clinical prejudices are rewritten as scientific understanding. Through medicalization of alternative etiologies, medical science remains a closed system.

Finally, medicalization imparts a moralistic tone to health-education practice. The script supplied by medical science constructs the role of the health educator very tightly. This is painful to health educators who identify with their audiences and are not inclined to reduce people to their compliance characteristics. Like anthropologists, health educators often desire to advocate for the communities and people they study.

Such desires notwithstanding, it is extremely difficult for health educators to escape from the worldview of medical science. In the official view of health-education campaigns such as Project CAN-DO, local cancer etiologies, through a process of medicalization, are seen only as symptoms of fatalism and denials of objective risk. As such, these health beliefs are material for a construction of a negative other, and are part of what makes the "hard to reach" population inscrutable (see Said 1978).

ANTHROPOLOGICAL PRACTICE

As I became more settled in my position at Fox Chase, I began to take more time to follow my own research interests. In my second year on the project, I worked on a survey on nutrition. On the survey form, I left a space where respondents could check a box if they were willing to be contacted for an in-depth interview. With this sample in hand, I planned a series of interviews. Using the demographic and attitudinal data from the survey forms, I chose potential respondents who represented a variety of ethnic backgrounds and a variety of viewpoints on nutrition and health. I supplemented this list by recruiting respondents at various community events.

By this time, I was familiar enough with my topic, and with how people spoke about it, to draw up a good list of questions. My list was brief. I decided to begin with a set of questions about heart disease, followed by identical questions about cancer. As noted above, the Project CAN-DO baseline survey had suggested a sharp contrast in community attitudes toward these two diseases; although my purpose was not to focus on the contrast per se, I thought it would make an interesting beginning. My questions about the two diseases were simple: "What comes to mind when you think about heart disease (cancer), the disease itself?" "Can you explain your own idea of what goes on inside the body with heart disease (cancer)?" "How would you explain this to someone twelve years old?" I also planned to ask about a character I refer to as "the defiant ancestor," who will be described below. Other than this, the interviews were entirely unstructured, except for a relatively simple set of questions, asked at the very end, concerning dietary habits.

At first, the interviews seemed to illustrate and pull together things I already knew. Read literally, the transcripts spoke of fatalism and of disagreement with the views of medical science. As I began, both as a health educator and as an anthropologist, to set the interviews in the context of all my Project CAN-DO experiences, however, I began to see that what my respondents said was part of a more complex discourse.

The following discussion is based on analysis of transcripts from twenty-five interviews and eight focus groups. The interviews were conducted by myself; the focus groups were conducted by other project staff members, although I was present at several. The interview respondents were all women; the focus groups include three groups of women, one group of men (with a male facilitator), and four mixed groups. The interview respondents were in their twenties, thirties, and forties. Many of the focus-group respondents were older. In all this material, as in my own informal notes about comments made at community meetings, women and men express similar views. Both my data and my experience leave me unsure as to whether there are differences in viewpoint according to age.

The major themes touched on in the transcripted material are described below. I will begin with a simple content analysis and move on to wider issues. (This research is also reported in Balshem 1991a.)

Lifestyle and Environment

Factors mentioned by interview and focus-group respondents as being preventive or causal for cancer, heart disease, or both are listed in Table 3. Following a schema presented by Pill and Stott (1985), I have classified them as environmental (extrapersonal) or lifestyle factors. Environmental factors (185 mentions) are mentioned more often than lifestyle factors (92 mentions) in regard to prevention and causation of cancer. The opposite pattern is seen for heart disease, with 47 mentions of lifestyle factors and only 13 mentions of environmental factors.

A respondent-by-respondent analysis of the interviews, excluding the focus groups, shows the same pattern. With regard to cancer, environmental factors are more readily brought to mind than lifestyle factors. Every interview respondent mentioned at least one environmental factor as being related to cancer prevention or causation, with an average of three such factors per respondent. In contrast, lifestyle factors were mentioned by only sixteen respondents as being causal or preventive for cancer. Seven more respondents mentioned lifestyle factors—notably smoking and diet—only to negate or express doubt about their link to cancer (these mentions are not included in Table 3). In contrast, with regard to the cause of heart disease, the respondent-

Table 3. Factors Mentioned as Preventing or Causing Cancer or Heart Disease: Twenty-five Interviews and Eight Focus Groups

Factors	Cancer	Heart Disease
Lifestyle Factors		
Diet	36	24
Smoking	19	8
Attitude	9	0
Proper exercise	5	7
Exposure to sun	6	0
Alcohol	4	4
Regular checkups	5	2
Taking care of self	4	0
Caffeine	0	2
Other lifestyle factors	4	0
Total mentions	92	47
Environmental (Extra-personal) Factors		
Environmental pollution	67	1
Heredity	38	8
Fate/God's will	18	0
Food additives	14	0
Cannot prevent	13	0
Causes not known	9	1
Occupational exposure	8	0
Stress	6	3
Everything causes	5	0
Germs	2	0
Other environmental factors	5	0
Total mentions	185	13

Source: After Table 1 in Balshem 1991a:157; the figures presented here reflect the addition of five more focus groups to the data set.

by-respondent analysis shows, again, an emphasis on lifestyle factors. Of the seventeen respondents who mention lifestyle or environmental factors as causal for heart disease, fourteen mention lifestyle only, three mention environment only, and four mention both.

Although my questions and probes for heart disease and cancer were identical, respondents talked at greater length about cancer. This is reflected in Table 3 in the greater absolute numbers of factors mentioned as being related to cancer.

Respondent discussions of cancer and heart disease are very different in emotional tone. Each interview respondent was asked, first for heart disease and then for cancer, the following question: "When I say [heart disease (cancer)], what does it make you think of?" Following is a representative set of answers, from one respondent, for heart disease and cancer, respectively:

The disease, you know, affects the blood stream. The vessels. I mean, it just taxes the heart, which is a muscle, and it just gets weak. You know. And it can't perform the job that it's supposed to do. As good as it's supposed to do it.

Oh, God, I have this terrible thought of cancer—it's like this great big thing that's eating up your whole insides. This big black thing. I just think of it as black. This big black thing that just goes along like a pac-man gobbling up your insides. . . . The movie *The Blob,* remember the blob would eat stuff and kept getting bigger and bigger. Well, that's kind of how I think of cancer. This great big blob of stuff that keeps increasing.

To this respondent, as to fourteen others, heart disease is a matter of mechanics gone wrong. Respondents may express that they themselves do not know how heart disease works, but they see it as a matter of finite knowledge. Heart-disease prevention, as well, is seen in straightforward terms. These quotes are typical:

Heart disease . . . say, you're okay, you're smoking, right? First of all, that takes away the oxygen, right? Then you've got the obesity with the cholesterol. That's going to clog your arteries. That's going to cause, you know, damage to the heart, little by little by little.

I never really read up on it. . . . I would just say the heart isn't as strong as yours or mine are. And because of the problem that the heart has, it's working harder and—and at times the heart just can't be working hard all the time. That's how I would put it.

Respondents express an easy acceptance of what they perceive as standard scientific knowledge concerning heart disease. The use of a mechanical model is expressive of the faith that these respondents have in the ability of modern medical science to understand heart disease fully. Regarding the prevention and cause of heart disease, respondents make fifteen value-neutral statements describing bodily mechanics—high blood pressure, clogged arteries, bad valves, and the like.

The use of the mechanical model, and the faith in medical science that it implies, is not seen in respondent discussion of cancer. No respondent made straightforward mechanical-model statements regarding the cause and prevention of cancer. Following is a typical answer to the question: "Cancer—what does it make you think of?": "Death. Because most of the time when you have cancer you wind up dead, you know. I know there's treatment and all but in my opinion I think of death."

Questions about cancer, unlike questions about heart disease, evoke answers that touch on universal mysteries. Here, as is typical, the respondent lowers her voice as she starts to speak about cancer, and comes without hesitation to the topic of death.

Fate is another topic often linked to cancer. Here, one respondent speaks of fate in relation to cancer and death: "If that person dies, it was—you know—that was—it was meant to be that that person would die with that disease. Where you—say you get two people maybe with the same kind where one will pull through, the other one won't."

Likewise, the following respondent speaks to the general issue of fate and disease control: "This area, that's pretty much the way people are brought up, you know, that you can try to cheat death but it's going to happen sooner or later, so—if it's your day to die and you don't get died one way you're gonna walk in front of a car and get hit and killed anyway."

Statements about fate are usually expressed with conviction, as counterpoints to my presumed advocacy of lifestyle theories of the causes of cancer. Respondents perceive, quite accurately, that their views are in opposition to scientific views, in which lifestyle is awarded center stage. Respondents do not, however, express a simplistic rejection of the relevance of lifestyle. They usually speak of fate as one factor of many, but one that is more powerful than lifestyle. The following respondents express this:

I think it's everything you eat and you do and a little bit from up there. . . . if you probably weigh everything out—I don't think you'll ever beat it. I do believe your time is when it is, too.

But no, I really in my heart, think that everything that, they're doing, we're learning, we're saying through education, whatever, is fine. Really. And you should follow, you should try to follow it. Okay? But I still feel that if you're gonna, you know, there's nothing you can do about it. I think it's God's will, that's all. I really do.

Talking about cancer carries us into issues of control over health in ways that talking about heart disease does not. Respondents stress lifestyle choices as factors causing heart disease, but they stress environmental forces when speaking of cancer. In discussion of cancer, respondents speak freely and at length of death and fate; discussions of heart disease are more mundane, often touching on mechanical models that indicate faith in the medical establishment's knowledge of the disease. Both the tone and content of respondent discourse reflect a more negative underlying attitude toward cancer.

I just think it's God's will, to tell you the truth, that's my personal opinion because, as I said, this is being a cancerous area and there's people living here and you know, and just their daily life, I guess, you know, their routine, but one might eat good and one might eat bad, one might smoke, one might not smoke, and it's still comin' up, you get it or you don't get it.

It's probably a lot easier with heart disease because like if you got maybe scar tissue on the heart—okay, they can remove that. Or in the vein—they could cut that part out and they could connect something else. Um—[*silence*]—you know, with cancer—I mean, that's so—[*silence*]—totally like the end of everything.

At least with your heart, if you take care of yourself and do what you're supposed to do, you'll be all right, but cancer—there's no control for it. No matter what you do, it's still there. . . . It's just—you bide your time—until, until—you know, until you die.

Science and Authority

Clearly, talking about cancer brings out feelings of resistance to scientific authority. In all the interview and focus-group transcripts, there are thirty-six direct denials of the scientific view of cancer prevention, with eighteen mentions of smoking and eleven mentions of diet as factors not associated with cancer. In contrast, standard knowledge concerning heart disease is not questioned by any respondent.

The following illustrate the common skepticism about the link between cancer and lifestyle, with regard to smoking:

I don't think cigarettes really gives you cancer—I haven't heard of a lot of people who got cancer from smoking, because people who don't smoke gets cancer of the throat. So you know, you can't say it's smokers that's going to get it when nonsmokers also get it. So it can't just come from that.

But then how about the people that don't smoke? Like my mother, like I told you, never smoked a day in her life. Why did she die of lung cancer? [MB: Well, why do you think she did?] Beats me. I have no idea, no idea. Wish I knew.

This may be read as a simple contradiction of a scientific message: that smoking and other lifestyle factors cause cancer. But also involved is a rejection of a perceived metamessage: that scientists know definitively what causes cancer. Associated with this is a critique of scientific authority for wrongly discounting the activity of powers beyond their ken.

Respondents express anger, frustration, and even disdain in reaction to the perceived arrogance of the scientist. On one hand, goes the discourse, science tells us that everything in our environment causes cancer; and on the other, it says that we can prevent cancer through changes in our lifestyle:

Every time you turn, like, no matter what you listen to—TV, radio, what have you, all right—this causes cancer, that causes cancer—you know what I mean? So, like, you know, like, all right, I opened my eyes this morning, I just breathed in twenty-nine gallons of cancer. You know what I mean? So, like, just opening your eyes, you're saying, "hello, cancer."

Or fluorocarbons in hair spray. Right? You got fluorocarbons in hair spray—you're gonna kick the bucket! Well, for eighteen years I was breathing in fluorocarbons, I must be ready to go at any time now. You know? Then they finally took it out. Or, "hair dye will give you cancer." Well, then I must have it. I mean definitely I'm a goner. I don't know when, but I must be a goner because of all these things that they had in there and nobody never told you they weren't any good.

In the following interchange, from the all-male focus group, one participant criticizes another for being too health conscious:

You're afraid of eating this and afraid of doing this, afraid of cancer, afraid of asbestos, and all that nonsense. My God, I went to a grammar school— I'm sure that the pipes must have leaked asbestos for all the six, seven years I was there. [A second participant:] Ah, that explains it! [*General laughter*] [A third participant:] Brain damage!

The sarcastic tone, commonly heard, only thinly veils the message— that scientists do not really know what causes cancer. Other respondents deliver this message straightforwardly, with a lively sense of challenge to the interviewer.

Over the last two decades everything has been this causes cancer and that— and people are to the point now where they think everything you eat causes cancer and nobody really knows what causes cancer.

This anger feeds into a wider stream of distrust. Expressed by four interview respondents, for instance, is the view that a cure for cancer is being withheld: "If you want my honest opinion, I think there is a cure for cancer. I believe deep down there is a cure, but it's the almighty buck again." In this view, the public is victimized by the medical establishment and the government, who conspire to maintain a profitably high level of cancer morbidity.

Talking about cancer draws us into images of victimization. For three interview respondents, and participants in two of the four focus groups, nuclear holocaust is an appropriate image for a victimized world (compare Sontag 1977). The following quotations are drawn from the focus groups:

[First respondent:] You know, it's really a contradiction. Life today. You know? It really is. . . . Everybody's out to scare you. I think that's why people you know, maybe take the negative attitude, because they think, "God, everybody's just out to," you know. [Second respondent:] Everybody's out to get you, no matter what you do, so just enjoy what you do and how you do it. [Facilitator:] Why do you think everyone's out to get you? What is it, what is it about the way things are? [First respondent:] I think the world in general. The peace and the war and this one fighting that one. When we grew up, we—we had the—the raids—the air raid tests where we would hide under the desks . . . now you've got nuclear—where—forget it! You ain't gonna be there!

No matter whether every person in the United States pickets against the nuclear bomb, if these people in Washington want it, they're gonna do it. You know, and if they want to push the button, they're gonna push it. So you feel like you don't have the control. . . . [Facilitator: What do you have control over in your life?] . . . I think you have control over your family. That part. I don't think you'll ever have control over your government or your health, you know, and anything like that.

This respondent sees her chances of gaining control over her health as being in a class with her chances of gaining control over her government. From a modern-day citizen of the United States, this is a very pessimistic assessment.

The following passage, from an interview, weaves many issues together:

It's the same way with the world and world peace and everything. We try, we pray, we talk, we sit down, but there's still that fear in everyone's heart that somebody's gonna push the button. . . . So who controls everything, you know. No matter what we do . . . if you don't eat the proper diet, if you do smoke, if you do drink, and . . . you run your body to the ground, it's gonna catch up with you a lot *sooner* than maybe the person who does everything, that eats all the right things and exercises and doesn't smoke and gets out, you know—but the ironic thing about it, he's the one who drops dead before the guy that's abusing everything! . . . . I don't think you control it. And if you're raised and . . . born to the faith that we are, you don't control it. Okay? He might let us think we do, but we don't. Why do babies die? Why are there crib deaths? . . . Why anything? It's just the way it is. You're not gonna change it.

Control, fate, and victimization—these are issues into which talking about cancer leads. Resentment of the authority of science is central. In many instances, statements about this issue carried such emotional force that they effectively brought my questioning to a halt.

A Minion of Fate

From the discourse of these community residents, one may glean an integrated structure of belief concerning the essential nature of cancer. This view of the nature of the disease is fundamentally different from that propounded by scientific medicine.

According to this view, cancer is at the same time "within us all" and "all around us." We are all born with it, and it can be activated by nearly anything—from a serious trauma, such as a major accident, to the most incidental of life events, such as a bump on the breast. It can also be activated by stress, which can mean the wearing effect of everyday living or of an especially difficult period of time. Substances present in the air, earth, and water can also activate it. The causes of cancer are everywhere. Once activated, cancer is invariably fatal. "Everything to me is cancerous, because it seems like every time you turn around, it causes cancer, I mean, you hear on TV, I mean, you touch somethin' and it might cause cancer." "I think we're all born with cancer cells, and I think certain things, maybe diseases or the environment, bring them out." The following, from the husband of an interview respondent, adds a male voice: "I'm a firm believer anyways that everybody has that [cancer] in their system. I really believe that, that everybody has something in their system. It just takes something else to trigger it off. . . . It's environmental. Something environmental triggers it off. It has to."

Descriptions of the cancer disease process suggest purposefulness and motivation. Cancer does more than simply grow: it takes over, hits your brain, burns you up, kills you from the inside out. The dominant metaphor (used by ten of the twenty-five interview respondents) is that cancer eats away at the body. It is spoken of as active, powerful, and impossible to stop: "Literally, the cancer is eating away the rest of the body—the rest of the cells in the body." "It just eats you up, I guess. It just starts and it doesn't stop, you know. . . . you always hear of it startin' and that they—it doesn't help, you know, some you hear on TV, they get cured but . . . it just goes and it doesn't stop."

Cancer is spoken of as a "sneaky disease," suggesting that the activity of the disease is capricious: "Like one day you could be fine and then turn around and you have cancer and it eats away at you." "It's a sneaky disease. . . . because it doesn't show itself. . . . There's cancer cells in everybody's body. Somewhere."

Cancer is also known as "the devil's disease," suggesting cruelty and evil as part of its nature. Following is an excerpt from a memorial article in a community newspaper:[2] "She was stricken by the devil's disease, cancer, and for 4 years she fought the disease till she had no more strength to fight, she died peacefully only after she was assured we could accept her death."

As with most minions of fate, cancer may punish those who notice or defy it. To think about cancer, to try to prevent it, is to tempt fate. Cancer testing is "looking for trouble." There is a hesitancy to speak the word *cancer* out loud. Like many others, community residents often refer to cancer as "The Big C" and are reluctant to be near cancer patients or speak to them about their disease. Sometimes, the word will not even be spoken within the larger family circle of a dying patient. One respondent spoke of her mother's death: "I don't know if she knew she had cancer. We never talked about it, we never did. But she wasn't stupid, she watched TV, she worked with people. I'm sure, you know, trying to protect us that she didn't discuss it."

Many community residents, then, speak of cancer as a purposeful entity that is capricious, cruel, and evil. The workings of cancer are workings of fate, and fate explains why one person rather than another falls ill. Cancer is a bad fate, in the face of which our bodies are permeable, affording us no protection within the physical and moral world. Because of cancer, our bodies contain and are tied to a force greater than the individual body and are not subject to individual control. The fear of cancer is the fear of annihilation, the fear of death.

Challenging fate is a risky business. Cancer inspires not challenge but taboo: "[Cancer is] taboo. Don't talk about it. If I don't talk about it, you know, or hear about it, I might not get it. You know?"

Defiance as Prevention

These statements of belief lead into statements about cancer prevention far different from those approved by scientific medicine. For one thing, everyone is vulnerable, regardless of personal habits. This vulnerability is so complete that making lifestyle changes to lower cancer risk is seen as useless:

I figure I can watch what I'm eating, and do this and do that, but yet I can still get cancer anytime. Anybody can, no matter what you do you still can get it, cause it doesn't matter what you do or whatever, if it's there, it's there.

I don't think you'll meet anyone who isn't—somewhere isn't going along with the new ideas of not—or cutting down smoking or not smoking or changing food habits . . . but I still feel strongly that . . . if you're gonna get it, you're gonna get it. And there's nothing we can do about it.

No matter what you do—if it's there, it's there. People who even have different lifestyles can get the same kind of cancer. So—either way, you know—if you're going to get it, I think you're going to get it, and that's it.

Can cancer, then, be prevented at all? An answer emerges at various places in the discourse but can be seen most clearly in stories about the defiant ancestor. The defiant ancestor, a golden age figure of the grandparental or parental generation, is often invoked by community residents during informal discussion periods after health education programs. The figure was introduced by eight out of twenty-five interview respondents, and it was recognized eagerly by others if I introduced it.

The defiant ancestor, so goes the story, smoked two packs of cigarettes a day, ate nothing but lard and bread, never went to the doctor, and lived until the age of ninety-three. The natural question that follows—and that followed during the interviews—is: what do you think these people did right? Why do you think they lived so long?

Above all else, defiant ancestors are hard workers. Physical labor, at work and at home, was the backbone of their existence: "That woman ever since I was born worked and worked and worked . . . woke up 4:30 every morning, did some wash, went to work, came home—she just went—and I think a lot of people, that keeps them going."

The defiant ancestor does not dwell on disease. Keeping a positive attitude is an important part of staying healthy; refusing to acknowledge symptoms is a way of keeping sickness at bay. Working hard and staying active are the best medicines:

That was on I think television the other day when they were saying that—I think it was a nurse talking and she said that the people that say, "Oh, my God! I'm afraid I might have cancer! I might have cancer!" They—they're the ones that tend to get it, more so than the ones that say, "Whatever's wrong with me, I'm going to fight it and I'm going to be strong!"

If you're the type of people that just sit around all the time, you're gonna be sick a lot. If you get up and move and go out and do things, they don't seem to be as sick that often. . . . [The old people] get up at five in the morning and go to bed at nine at night and they work all the time.

If a person thinks—feels that they're going to get sick, they do get sick. And—because they have that in their mind . . . Myself, I just take one day at a time, and I don't look at what's going to happen tomorrow because tomorrow might not come.

Many respondents state proudly that they themselves have many of the attributes of these defiant ancestors. This is particularly common among the men, who tend, perhaps, to talk a little bit less about fate and a lot more about being tough. The following quotations, from the all-male focus group, illustrate this:

If you hit me, it'll put a dent in your car. That's why I don't think there's a lot of people who are really concerned about health concerns. . . . So far as

I'm concerned, I'm healthy, and I'm not going—going to do anything to change it.

Yeah, if I had to attribute anything to my father's death—it was not doing anything after he retired. In other words, losing interest, you know, not keeping involved with things, walks and all. In other words, it's like a machine—you allow it to get rusty and it slows down. I think.

Positive thinking can help you be cured of cancer.

Part of not dwelling on sickness is staying away from the doctor, ignoring medical advice, and refusing medications:

You've got to stop and think about these people. They're of the old school, I think, and they know how to work hard. . . . They came over—they worked like horses. They were strong, and I think—years ago, people didn't run to a doctor. They had the old remedies.

My grandmother, she doesn't, she never went to the doctor's until the last couple months, she was in so much pain that she went, she has an ulcer and you know, and they thought maybe she had something like Reagan had [colon cancer]. . . . But it took her until she was in *that much* pain to go.

Working hard and toughing it out—it is a point of pride to delay going to the doctor until you are nearly dysfunctional. Hiding sickness is also prized:

I would feel that even though if I'm going to die, I'd rather do it longer instead of dying sooner; and making myself happy and the people around me happy so it doesn't even think that I'm dying. Just let it just go my normal life and just be happy and just don't even pay attention that I'm going to die, just keep it going as long as I can.

Even when diagnosed with cancer, those who follow the old ways can show themselves to have resources that medical science does not understand. This story, echoed by others, shows an ancestor who was defiant even in the face of death:

Like my father—he had leukemia, which is cancer of the blood. They told him that he only had two months to live, and he says, "No way—I'm makin' that summer because I'm going to my boat." And the doctors still can't believe to this day that he made four months. . . . And he died at the end of September. So I think outlook has a lot to do with it. If you make up your mind you're going to do something about it, you can. . . . He was a fighter.

Through discourse about the defiant ancestor, respondents express a theory of cancer prevention that is consistent with their expressed view of the disease. If cancer is a minion of fate, then escaping the notice of fate is preventive medicine. An expression of evil purpose— one that seeks to victimize us—is warded off by a positive attitude, by which we refuse to allow evil to overwhelm us. Cancer is also capricious, irrational, striking regardless of direct efforts to control it. Are such efforts, then, counterproductive, serving to challenge forces that we hope will ignore us? The defiant ancestor suggests that dwelling on cancer prevention is foolish. The following interview respondent expresses a common ultimate assessment:

I feel that even if you're healthy and you don't go to the doctor's you still—you know, you still can live, and even if you smoke and all, you still can live until an age. So it doesn't matter what you do, you still die when your time comes. So it doesn't matter if you change your diet, or stop smoking, when your time's up it's up and there ain't nothin' you can do about it. But 'least they lived to be happy and did what they wanted to do. That's the more important thing.

And the following exchange, from the all-male focus group, adds more than a pinch of local humor:

I—I think one of the curses of our society is, is a media that, um—tells us all these things that are bad for us, and then six months later somebody else does a research study that says, "Oh, no, that's not too bad. Cholesterol— you *need* cholesterol. Boy, you'd better get a good supply of cholesterol." That's the latest, you know. So now the—you know, now the media comes out—*The New England Journal of Medicine*, you know, is the greatest source of—of all this stuff. You know, it all comes out of there. So one time you're bad, the next time you're good. So nobody pays attention after a while because there's too many—too much conflict. Nobody knows. [Second participant:] Just remember one thing: sex won't rot your teeth. [First participant:] Well, it depends on how you do it. [*Laughter*]

Cancer, Control, and Causality

In the river wards, talking about cancer can mean talking about fate. This may be seen literally, as a reflection of beliefs that are more or less heartfelt, depending on the person and the circumstances. But another understanding of this talk may be drawn from looking at wider contexts.

Most community residents express a different set of beliefs about cancer causation, and causation in general, than that propounded by science. The causal universe they describe is one in which God and luck weave mysterious and unpredictable connections, endangering us all in sometimes purposeful ways. Etiologies that reside within this cosmos allow for specific diseases or occasions of disease to be described as more or less tied to the purposes of fate. For cancer, the tie is seen as being generally strong. The path to survival and cancer prevention in an unpredictable universe is to avoid, focus elsewhere, and persevere.

But to some extent, the meaning of such talk is to be understood by reading it as performance. This talk confronts the health educator as critical talk about the authority of science. And science, according to this talk, cannot see past the end of its own nose. In this community discourse, connections such as that between food and general health are held to coexist with other mechanisms that science would render invisible. Scientists, so goes the critique, see a partial view of the world. What is more, they are too arrogant to admit the reality of anything not within reach of their imagined powers of control.

Community residents invoke the moral authority of their ancestors and see that invocation as creating an irrefutable stance within the discourse. Behind this stance is more than a logically consistent position regarding the best way to avoid cancer. The defiant ancestor also embodies community lifeways, self-reliance, and defiance of scientific medical advice. The ancestors confront us to say that in local health cosmology, science has not yet exorcised the power or the value of tradition.

Community residents are aware that the worldview they express is regarded by science as a problem, as a view that needs changing. Scientists, in the residents' interpretation, see themselves as possessing the only valid authority, one that dictates a negating of the value of deep-seated wisdoms. The antagonism that the urban working class feels toward scientific authority is tied into a larger antagonism toward powerful forces from the outside that bear down upon the community like a juggernaut, causing social, economic, and health problems that are beyond local control. In this context, local traditions are held up, to self and other, as being of higher value than scientific knowledge. For residents of this high-cancer-risk community, excluding external views about cancer is important.

Low control over life circumstances is central in working-class experience, in contrast to the experience of higher status persons, such as scientists, physicians, and health educators.[3] This is clearly felt, by community residents, with regard to the control of knowledge about cancer. Community residents have less connection, or hope of finding a connection, to the systems by which health professionals access, control, and create information that is accorded scientific legitimacy. They are keenly aware that their chances of influencing public policy on health research are very low. They experience their exclusion from power on many levels, from the official disregard of their views to the inability of residents to prevent the profound pollution of their air, water, and workplaces.

Thus, the community expression of a counterpoint to science is tied to strong feelings about access to power in society. From the community residents comes a disinclination to accept their assigned position as "targets" of a health education campaign. They have seen themselves labeled as sick, and they turn this around to label their social and material environment as sick. They have considered blaming themselves as victims and have rejected the notion. Scientific authority, clearly, does not consider their interpretations of experience to be valid. So they use rhetoric about fate as a shield, and charge the scientists with being guilty of hubris.

THE ANTHROPOLOGIST'S VIEW

My own view begins with the dramatic contrast between the silence of the public audience and the eagerness of the furtive invitations into community homes. The public audience was sullen; the interviews radiated with fun and excitement. Do the public and private discourses relate to the same commentary?

To understand that they do, one must remember the different contexts in which they occur. Public forums such as health-education programs belong to scientific and educational authority. The scientist (health educator) lectures, and the audience listens, with pastor and school principal present. In this context, community residents assume the rebellious stance of the disempowered and alienated student. This stance—an expression of what Willis calls the "counter-school culture" (1977:2)—is central to and familiar in working-class life (also compare Freire 1971). In this way, they enact resistance to the position they feel they are put in, through their wider social disenfranchisement, by powerful authorities such as that of science. Concretely, they look bored.

The teasing and sotto voce hinting that go on after the presentation are a challenge to the health educator to get down off the stage and listen. This is shown clearly, for instance, by the teasing that I received about eating an offered piece of cake. We know you eat cake just like we do, the teasing says, and that you only assume that superior role while standing on the stage. Come down, and we will respond to your lecture.

In contrast, the kitchen, the site of most of the interviews, belongs to the community. There, residents were at last emboldened, transformed into respondents with a purpose. In my view, most saw their interview as an opportunity to enact a performance, to assume a rhetorical stance, in front of a representative of science. In a rare happening, a scientist had made an appearance in the community. More rare still, she had signaled a lowering of interpersonal barriers and asked to come into community homes. This created an opportunity to express a treasured local value—one expressed internally quite often, on the front stoop or in front of the television, but seldom in the actual presence of a scientist. Through the interviews, respondents lived the drama of speaking their views to the outside, to the adversary, who, in a delicious reversal of the usual power mechanisms in the medical encounter, was herself in a position of special vulnerability. Yet, the interviews did not have an adversarial feel—perhaps because respondents did not see the agreement of the interviewer as important.

Both public and private responses of the community to their health educators may be seen as what James C. Scott has termed everyday forms of resistance. Scott describes such resistance as "the ordinary weapons of relatively powerless groups: foot dragging, dissimulation, false compliance, pilfering, feigned ignorance, slander, arson, sabotage, and so forth" (1985:29).

The more opaque of these methods—false compliance, feigned ignorance—have often been read as peasant fatalism and resistance to innovation. Indeed, as Scott tells us, early views of the intellectual life of subordinate classes portrayed them as strongly constrained on the level of thought by the processes of hegemony. Scott describes the views of Antonio Gramsci, the Italian revolutionary socialist: "By creating and disseminating a universe of discourse and the concepts to go with it, by defining the standards of what is true, beautiful, moral, fair, and legitimate, [those in power] build a symbolic climate that prevents subordinate classes from thinking their way free" (Scott 1985:39).

Scott's portrait of lived experience in a peasant village, of everyday practice in a subordinate class environment, however, supports the argument that hegemony is not an omnipotent process. On the contrary, control of the terms of discourse, the definers of value and belief, is the focus of a potent struggle. Likewise, in the community described here, the struggle is a potent one. The maintenance of a rebellious consciousness is part of the construction of valued self, valued community, valued life, in a subordinate class environment. Self and community, valuing and supporting each other, process myriad insults, betrayals, and frustrations. Local belief and tradition is asserted as superior, as is local insight into the workings of authority and hegemony. Community residents assert local control of the value ascribed to local tradition. With regard to beliefs about cancer, these assertions are made in the context of powerfully emotional issues surrounding fate, suffering, life, and death. What is being negotiated is control: control of local belief and activity regarding cancer, control and causality.

Resistance, of course, is also not omnipotent (again, see Scott 1985; also see discussion in Rebel 1989). The negotiation of powerlessness demands that we realize things in certain contexts that we do not realize in others. The data presented here show a critique of the construction of medical knowledge, but one that is specifically expressed—and perhaps specifically realized—through talking about cancer. When these same respondents talk about heart disease, they express a "routine compliance" (Scott 1985:278–84) with dominant medical models.[4]

For residents of Tannerstown, talking about cancer opens up a specific text, one that contains an overt and elaborate analysis of dominance and control. There are a number of reasons why this is so.

First, there is the material nature of the disease. As Susan Sontag (1977) so eloquently tells us, and as the material here illustrates, the cancer disease process serves as an apt metaphor for loss of control. Beliefs focusing on cancer as uncontrollable have been documented among middle-class people and among working-class African Americans in the United States; beliefs about cancer being uncontrollable, mysterious, and fatal have been recorded in Australia, Britain, France, Israel, Italy, Japan, and Quebec.[5] Patterson (1987) shows the presence of such beliefs in the United States in the 1800s. This consistency may be related to commonalities in the bodily experience of most cancers.

Second, loss of control is an important issue for the postindustrial working class. They are not alone in this: it is an important issue for all of us in the postmodern world (Lipset and Schneider 1983; Newman 1989; Reich 1987), and, according to Sontag, acts generally to amplify the dread of cancer. But for traditionally patriotic, poor inner-city whites, the issue is highlighted by the current decline of their class and country, the fading of glory days. This puts in context the general tendency for groups of lower socioeconomic status in the United States to exhibit a special resistance to scientific views on and recommendations for cancer control.[6]

But to understand fully the meaning of cancer in Tannerstown, one must look at local conditions. Living with high cancer mortality, and with smokestacks and waste dumps, fuels a specific penetration of scientific and medical hegemony, one that resonates with the wider political issue of low control. Tannerstowners witness a lot of cancer, and a high percentage of those who have cancer do not seek medical attention until the disease is at a late stage. Too often, they then proceed through agonizing suffering to an early death. Thus, ironically, Tannerstowners feel special resentment toward medical advice regarding the prevention, early detection, and treatment of cancer. Such advice blames individuals, where community statements of belief in fate would forgive them (compare Fortes 1987). Thus, advice to quit smoking, eat better, and go for regular checkups may suffer through association with the issue of cancer prevention.[7]

In sum, it is generally true, and particularly so from the vantage point of Tannerstown, that if one is thinking about control, cancer is good to think with. And control is the issue on which community thought about cancer has focused. The community situates the assumptions of scientific cancer control within a wider context of power and social class. This context is difficult for medical science to recognize. Scientific medicine is often spoken of as a closed system, one that cannot easily work with other points of view (see, for instance, Janzen 1978). In an important sense, what scientific medicine is closed to is an admission of the problematic nature of its own power.

The community critique is also concerned with the issue of causality—that is, with the paradigmatic tendency of science to delimit the causal universe to that which it says and sees. The community critique, as detailed above, defines this as hubris and posits an identity of body and spirit that can be expressed and understood only crudely from within the scientific paradigm.

It is no coincidence that the community critique of medical science mirrors that of critical studies in medical anthropology (compare

DiGiacomo 1992). As the authority of scientific medicine is increasingly challenged, similar critiques surface on many fronts, including that of a progressive consciousness within medicine itself (for instance, Aoun 1992; Hilfiker 1985; White 1988).

But beyond this interpretation of community discourse as critique lies a view of the discourse as a series of acts and thoughts of resistance. Through performance, the community turns the subject of the discourse around and defines the meaning of the discourse for itself. The residents see themselves being blamed as victims, targeted for education, and they reject it and respond with a critique of their own. Where we would make them the objects of scientific study, they make science the object of their own analysis. Thus, we must see not only how they are the subjects of our practice, but how we are the subjects of theirs.

A CANCER DEATH | 4 |

Have we reached such a point in our "health-conscious" society that every
individual who suffers an illness classified as "preventable" must bear the
burden of responsibility for that illness? Why isn't it possible to just get
sick without it also being your fault? . . . We seem to view raising a
cheeseburger to one's lips as the moral equivalent of holding a gun to
one's head.

Paul R. Marantz, "Blaming the Victim: The Negative Consequence
of Preventive Medicine," *American Journal of Public Health*,
October 1990

Like, they'll say he smoked and drank and that's why he got cancer. And
I'm trying to say all the research isn't right.

Jennifer, the patient's wife

In the previous chapter, I argued that in Tannerstown, public opposition to lifestyle theories of cancer causation resonates with overtly
political resistance to powerful external forces. Here, I will trace a
replaying of the same opposition in a clinical setting. The medical
case history I will discuss involves the death of a Tannerstown man
with metastatic pancreatic cancer. The conflicts involved are common in clinical oncology and may be experienced between physicians
and patients of any social background. But in this case, as in the
community setting, the issues are presented in an elaborately insightful and unusually outspoken way by a Tannerstowner, the wife of the
patient.

This medical case history is more than the story of a cancer death. It
is also the story of a dispute between a Tannerstown woman and her
husband's physicians. This dispute was probably not experienced co-
herently as such by any one of the many physicians involved in the
case. In the eyes of the patient's wife, however, the dispute is clear; it
concerns control of decisions, information, and the official record of
her husband's illness and death. The climax of the dispute occurs over

the issue of what is legitimately recognized, in the medical record, as the cause of his cancer and his death.

In constructing my narrative of this case, I have drawn on three texts: the retrospective narrative of the patient's wife; the written medical record, obtained, with permission, from the hospital in which the patient died; and general reflections, again retrospective, from one of the attending physicians on the case. This multiplicity of texts complicates the story and renders the characters as too complex to fit into easy analytical categories. In the end, only a multiplicity of readings will fully represent my view of the case.

PRESENTATION OF THE CASE

John, the name I will give to the patient in this case, died at the age of forty-two. The direct cause of his death was pneumonia; the antecedent cause was pancreatic cancer, metastatic to both lungs and to numerous other areas of the body. The main character in the story to follow is his wife, whom I shall call Jennifer.

I first met Jennifer four years after John's death, when she agreed to be interviewed for my study on local perceptions of Project CAN-DO. Over the next several years, I visited her on two more occasions. Between these visits and telephone conversations, I have spoken with her for more than ten hours.

When we first spoke, Jennifer lived in Tannerstown, where her family had lived for three generations. When she and John were first married, they had left the neighborhood. But several years later, her parents purchased a bar in the next neighborhood and moved to the apartment above the bar. Her mother, she told me, wanted her close by and offered her the house in Tannerstown. So Jennifer and John moved into the house that Jennifer had grown up in, and they raised their children there. Jennifer found that a lot of people her age had moved away from Tannerstown for a time but were now returning. Prices for housing elsewhere were sky high, and there was something missing in those other neighborhoods, anyway.

I think most of Tannerstown is family. . . . My aunt lives here. Oh, all my relatives lived here, but eventually they died off. My cousin lived on B Street. He just moved. He just moved this year, but he lived there while my kids were growing up. It's—the girl down the street, I know her mother-in-law. Lives a little ways away. So it's—the girl over there is cousins with the girl over here. [*Laughs*] But I like that. You know, I'll tell you—I like it. They really help me with my kids. If I want to go out or something, my kids know they can't party here because my neighbor has my key and if it gets too loud in here she's allowed to walk right in. . . . I don't even tell her. She just—as soon as she hears some banging, she runs in and says, "Don't you ruin this house! Your mother—" They are those type of people. . . . And even my dad, when they lived here, um, they shared everything. They said they remember the parties in their neighborhood. Just neighborhood parties, for a Friday night out. You didn't have money. So they said—he was the first one with a TV. So they used to come in here and watch TV. You know, it was that type of thing, years ago, see. And a lot of them remember my mom and dad, so they were really nice to me when I moved here.

At the time of his illness, John was employed at a metal-working plant located not far from Tannerstown. Photographs and family memories show a quiet family man, slightly built, with short blond hair and a kind expression.

Onset of Illness

Jennifer was an informant with an agenda. I began our first interview with my standard introductory questions. But when we got to the subject of cancer treatment, she began to tell her story.[1] (As noted earlier, my own comments are bracketed and identified with my initials, MB.)

I feel some of the hospitals are more educated than others. I didn't realize it at the time . . . but I think they should teach people because I know when my husband got sick, I knew nothing. I didn't even know where to go. And you know, if you hit the right doctor, I think you have—not a better shot—I think timing is what it is—but, uh, maybe you're more pleased, let's put it that way, with the results. And I hit a lot of wrong hospitals.

At the onset of his terminal illness, John was without a primary-care physician.

He just really didn't have a doctor. Well, he had one, but he died, which is ironic because the guy would have known him well enough, I think, to know that it wasn't his nerves. The new doctor felt it was his nerves. Yeah—and you get that all the time. [MB: Holy crow! Like sometimes if they don't know what it is, they might say that.] Well, I could see them believing it. Now I can. I thought it was his nerves. [MB: So he died of cancer?] Yeah. Yeah. I thought it was his nerves. My neighbor next door, being older, said she thought it was cancer. And she kept saying to me, "How's your husband? How's your husband?" I'd say, "Oh, God, he's being a pain in the ass this summer. I don't know what's wrong with him! He's not eating. He's not doing this—" You know. And of course, nobody wants to say an opinion, and I guess with age, you get to know or recognize things. Maybe she's seen people. I don't know. And then when everything came out, she said, "I had a feeling it was serious." She wasn't sure why, she said, but she'd known us like twelve years, and she said she saw him losing the weight so fast, and I didn't. [MB: Because you saw him every day.] I guess, yeah. And then when his friends saw him—they hadn't seen him for a while and we'd bump into them, people would look and say, "What the hell is wrong with you?" And then I'd start thinking, you know, as more people and more people approached you and said it, you know. And one day I—I had to really step back and look and I thought, "He is sick."

In late September, John developed diarrhea and began to vomit constantly. He was admitted to Hospital A, a fairly good community hospital, apparently as an emergency patient, and was put on intravenous therapy for rehydration. The physician they had gone to, who had originally diagnosed the problem as nerves, now wished the patient to have tests. But this physician did not have privileges at Hospital A, so John was transferred to Hospital B, a weaker institution. The following is from the Hospital B discharge summary:

This is a 42 year old Caucasian gentleman who was admitted with weight loss of about 10 lbs. since July of this year. He had abdominal pain preceded by right loin pain since June of this year. He had been vomiting for the last five days prior to admission and had diarrhea for the last two weeks. He was well until June of this year when he was . . . afflicted with pain in the right kidney region. He also had a muscle pull and trauma to the right lower chest and attributed this pain to that trauma. However, the pain continued and it moved to midabdominal region. He consulted the doctor at his place of work who was treating him for muscle pain. Then he went to his family physician who treated him with antacids, Ativan and Librax but this was to no avail. . . . PAST MEDICAL HISTORY: Positive for seizure disorder [seven years ago] for which he had extensive work-up but no treatment was prescribed. It was ascribed to possible alcohol intake. SOCIAL HISTORY: Smoked 1½ packs for the last 22 years and had not taken a drink in the last 3 or 4 months although he used to drink heavily in the past. . . . PHYSICAL EXAMINATION: . . . Diagnostic impression on admission was dehydration, vomiting, diarrhea, abdominal pain, weight loss, rule out malignancy, and rule out peptic ulcer disease. LAB DATA: . . . of note was the presence of questionable antigen CEA [carcinoembryonic antigen]. On 10/5 it was 22.4 and on 10/11 it was 31.7 and it was repeated and report was pending at the time of discharge. Urinalysis was normal on two occasions. Barium enema normal. Dorsal spine x-ray—no bony abnormality in the dorsal spine. Ultrasound of abdomen and kidney normal, limited visualization of the pancreas which was unremarkable. This pancreatic study was done twice and each time was reported as normal, no suggestion of any pancreatitis.

Ultrasounds and x-rays taken at Hospital B were read at Hospital C, a teaching hospital with better facilities. The relevance of this will be seen below.

From the time of John's admission, physicians at Hospital B considered the possibility that he might have cancer. The note to "rule out malignancy" indicates that they had planned further tests to rule out or possibly establish, if only through a process of elimination, a diagnosis of cancer. Also noted is the elevation of John's CEA level. The presence of this antigen in the bloodstream signals the possible presence of a malignancy. Usually, medical care in the United States would at that point involve open discussion with the patient regarding the probability of cancer. Appropriately, Jennifer's view of John's stay at Hospital B focuses on this issue of diagnosis. The questions that linger in her mind, years later, concern control of information. How much did they know? Did they diagnose him as having cancer? Did they do so and not tell her? Or not tell John? Or did John know and not tell her?

So he went to [Hospital B], and of course the tests take so long. He was in there about three weeks. Apparently—I don't know the whole story. Apparently, they must have said something to him, and he just wasn't saying anything to me. [MB: So they diagnosed him at (Hospital B)?] Nothing definite. Nothing said to me, but something must have been said to him. When I was talking to this doctor later, I said to him, "He has cancer." And he said, "I told him that." And of course I wasn't going to argue with my husband. He was sick then. And I didn't believe him. I said, "You couldn't have told him," I said, "because I think we're close enough—he would have told me." And he said, "I don't know what to tell you."

After three weeks, Jennifer decided to have her husband transferred to Hospital D, a small suburban hospital with limited resources, where he could be treated by her cousin's doctor. Their original primary physician questioned this: "He said—well, first he said, you know, 'Why are you transferring him?' I said, 'Well,' I said, 'I just think he has something,' I said, 'and you—' Plus, I was very upset."

The unfinished sentence marks a point at which Jennifer hesitates to verbalize, even now, the criticism she would level at this physician. Later, she describes her motive in seeking care from her cousin's physician: her cousin had described him as being easy to communicate with. This implies a finishing of her sentence: "I just think he has something," *and you are either not seeing it, or you are shutting me out of that knowledge.*

Another point of concern to Jennifer was the length of time it had taken for the results of the Hospital C radiology studies to be made available. To Jennifer's knowledge, the results were still not available after one week. It is not clear whether these results had in fact been known earlier to the Hospital B physicians, or to John, but they were not made known to Jennifer, who was trying to make informed decisions about her husband's care.

I was really upset because it was like over a week and they didn't get the x-rays. That's why I really had him transferred . . . over a week and they, nobody was getting any results back. So I just felt they were sort of pushing me off. You know, when we decided to transfer to [my cousin's] doctor, they told me to bring x-rays, I called [Hospital C] myself, told them the story and they said to me, "It usually takes us 24 hours to get x-rays together." Now, they could have had them in 24 hours. He said, "But—" I had like an 11 o'clock appointment. I called them at 9—he said, "I'll have them ready for you in an hour. Come down and get them." That's what I said to these other doctors: "Why do you do that—like when somebody's so sick?" I said, "Just—" I said, "Over a week you're telling me" . . . I said, "I would have picked them up for you," I said, "if that was the problem."

Jennifer's memory of her complaints to the Hospital B physicians is intense. "I said" is repeated after each phrase, as the emotional experience of having said these things is relived.

When she went to pick up John's studies from the radiology department at Hospital C, Jennifer met a person whom she identifies only as the "blood doctor."

That blood doctor, he was helping me get some of the x-rays together and when I was leaving he said to me, "Don't worry too much." He said, "I really don't think it's cancer." Well, then I thought they were all nuts. What the hell are they talking about? I still didn't think it was—and, just not being educated enough, I guess, I said—um, I just looked at him and thought he was nuts, although he said, "I think it's something with his liver."

The discharge summary for Hospital B shows a concern with the issue of liability, documenting that the patient had willingly and knowingly assumed full responsibility for the discharge:

Consultation with hematologist was also requested for elevated sedimentation rate and CEA and serum haptoglobin level was ordered along with the ultrasound of the abdomen, the latter two tests are pending at the time of discharge. However, the patient and the patient's family was insistent that the patient be discharged and followed as an outpatient because of financial strains and domestic reasons and therefore, the patient after being well informed of the consequences of his leaving the hospital and assuming the responsibility so that he has unfailing follow-up as an outpatient by the family physician, hematologist and myself, the patient was discharged.

The radiology report from Hospital C, dated the day after the patient's discharge, includes the following recommendation: "Ultrasound examination of the pancreas or specific CT [computerized tomography] examinations of the pancreas as indicated."

Diagnosis

At Hospital D, the diagnosis of cancer was quickly made clear to Jennifer.

Yeah—well, as soon as [Hospital D] saw him, two days, they said, "It's cancer." I said, "What?" I said, "These doctors had him for three, four weeks," I said, "and you're telling me in two days." Of course it could have advanced by then, but he said—I said, "How do you know when they didn't know?" They said, "Well, the symptoms are all there."

John underwent two surgical procedures at Hospital D: removal of a mass blocking the lower bowel; and partial removal of a mass encircling and invading the bones of the spine, which caused pain and muscular weakness in his legs.[2] Hospital D physicians assumed that the bowel was the primary site of John's cancer, and his treatment was consistent with this diagnosis.

By this time, Jennifer herself felt in need of medical care. She asked her husband's new primary physician, her cousin's physician, for medication. He refused her request, thereby gaining her respect, because to Jennifer, as to most Tannerstowners, toughing it out without drugs is a positive value.

I liked him. He wouldn't give me any medication so I liked him. Cause the one time, you know, I said to him, "You'd better give me something." And he said, "Get out of here," he said. "I've been watching you every day." He said, "You're driving too far. I just don't want you on medication." Because I said, "I can't eat." And he said, "That's your nerves." I said, "That's what they thought my husband had!" And he said, "Now don't go getting paranoid!" He said to me, "Really, it's your nerves, now."

Despite her personal satisfaction with this physician, she questioned the quality of care that her husband was receiving at Hospital D.

Now, [Hospital D] isn't too educated as far as medicine goes. He was zapped out there. He was hallucinating there. And they weren't—[MB: That's awful.] Oh, *was* it awful! My cousin and her husband came once and they walked out—they said—you know! So of course, then I thought, "God! Is this how he's going to be like the rest of his life? On this medication and stuff?" . . . I mean, I couldn't even stand seeing him then. He even said, when he came out of it, "I realized I was doing that stuff," and he said, "but I just couldn't stop myself," he said, "from doing it." One time he was collecting eggs from the ceiling, putting them in baskets. And my kids saw him like that. And my kids said—my one boy said to me, "I'm not going any more."

John was being treated for pain with large doses of methadone, Demerol, and Vistaril. He was hallucinating, and moreover, his pain was not well controlled.

With the diagnosis of cancer in the open, Jennifer faced a decision about one more transfer. Hospital D had sent her husband's tests to Hospital F, a major teaching hospital with an excellent oncology program, for review. Jennifer arranged to have her husband transferred to Hospital F, seeking state-of-the-art care for John. At the time of this transfer, she again had contact with the blood doctor at Hospital C, regarding transfer of her husband's records. He urged her to have John admitted to Hospital E, an institution that Jennifer had not considered. Hospital E is a strong community hospital with a good oncology program.

He said, because he just felt [Hospital E] was the best hospital then, not [Hospital F]—and that they would try harder, and they would work day and night with him. [MB: So—so then he was in (Hospital E)?] No, I just didn't know what to do at that point. I just already had arrangements for [Hospital F], so I said—I said, these doctors think I'm nuts the way it is—

so I said I—[MB: Well, what are you supposed to do? I mean, you have to go by what they're telling you.] Yeah, but in a way now, I wasn't happy—he told me I wasn't going to be happy with [Hospital F].

The State of the Art

In Jennifer's estimation, John received superior medical care at Hospital F. At the time of his admission, he was described as cachectic—that is, he appeared to be wasting away. He was still heavily medicated, in pain, and unable to walk.

He got to [Hospital F] and they said to me, "How long has he been like that?" I said, "Since his operation." They said, "It's the wrong medicine." So they brought their specialists in and the next day I couldn't *believe* the next day—then I thought a miracle was going to happen. The medication—they were more educated. As I'm saying, each hospital is *so* different. And it's terrible. Why don't they all get together and have meetings once a month and tell each other?

John's pain medication was changed to Dilaudid, with an almost immediate improvement in pain control. A social worker's note two days after admission gives us a rare glimpse of John himself:

Patient alert, oriented and articulate at time of visit. He appears mildly anxious and is somewhat focused on details of his medical history. . . . He states he and wife feel much more hopeful since change in medical care and definitive diagnosis of problems and that prior to that he was "hanging in there." Denied depression, anger, etc., but states he feels his problem would have been diagnosed much sooner if long-time family doctor was still alive. Patient described numerous incidents in which he diagnosed and "cured" family medical problems, indirectly expressing wish for same now.

This professional judgment entails a subtext of criticism. The patient is "somewhat focused" on the details of a medical history that would almost undoubtedly command anyone's focus; depression and anger are not simply absent, they are denied; and the social worker puts quotes around John's claim that his family doctor cured many illnesses, indicating her distance from what she sees as folk understandings and his naive faith that some doctors are better than others.

Five days after admission, Hospital F physicians had settled on the lung or the pancreas as likely primary sites for John's cancer, with metastases to the intestine and bone. Oat cell carcinoma of the lung was chosen as a working diagnosis. Appropriate chemotherapy was begun, along with intensive rehabilitation therapy to help John regain his ability to walk. After a nineteen-day stay, John was discharged "with a considerable decrease in his pain and a considerable increase in his ability to ambulate, and in a overall much improved status." Outpatient chemotherapy and radiation therapy were scheduled.

Notes from the social worker indicate that both the patient and his wife were coping well, although at one point it is noted that Jennifer "expresses fear about asking physicians for medical information, especially concerning lung involvement, as this threatens her hopefulness he will be okay."

Again, the social worker's note is loaded with interpretations. Who suggested that Jennifer's motivation is to protect her hopefulness— Jennifer, or the social worker? According to Jennifer, her difficulties in communicating with John's physicians about lung cancer are rooted more in the realities of physician-patient communication patterns than in her own internal psychological state. In any case, Jennifer was, as the blood doctor had predicted, unhappy with Hospital F. Her unhappiness was not with her husband's medical care but with the management of medical knowledge by Hospital F staff.

I wish I would have tried [Hospital E]. If I had it to do over again, I would have tried—if I was more educated and knew what hospitals did what. And I do think a study hospital—although [Hospital F] is a study hospital. But, uh, my idea there was—they were too smart. They were too smart. They didn't want to listen to people. . . . They got him off the medication. . . . That was the only thing I liked at [Hospital F]. The thing I didn't like there was, like I said, I think they're too educated.

"They were too smart"—"they're too educated." These are said with a low, intense tone, and an air of grim and final judgment.

Concerned about the Wrong Things

John spent the holidays at home and experienced some transient benefit from chemotherapy. After about six weeks, however, his general
condition had worsened dramatically, with an increase in pain. He was
readmitted to Hospital F for terminal care.

At this point, with the grave nature of John's illness clear and the
best possible medical care being pursued, the issue of making sense of
it came to a climax for Jennifer. Throughout John's illness, she had
struggled with issues relating to the control of medical information.
Now, she focused on the specific matter of the inclusion and exclusion
of information on John's medical chart. Her underlying concern was
control of the legitimate medical statement of the cause of John's
illness and impending death.

At issue was the following section of John's medical history, taken at
the time of his first admission to Hospital F and now appearing in
typewritten form in his chart:

PAST MEDICAL HISTORY: Remarkable for the questionable seizure, may have
been alcohol related, no known etiology and no further seizures [for the
past seven years]. . . . SOCIAL HISTORY: Patient is married, fairly extensive
history of alcohol abuse, none in the last several months. Also there is a 22
year history of cigarette smoking ($1\frac{1}{2}$ packs).

Through a staff indiscretion and a Tannerstown connection, Jennifer
was told that John's hospital chart identified him as an alcoholic. Medical charts are by law open to the patient and next of kin, but medical
practice at Hospital F, as at most hospitals, discourages patients and
their families from seeing them. Jennifer, however, was aware of her
rights and was determined to voice her challenge.

So I waited a couple days, and the one—the therapist had left it. So I was
looking through it and the doctor comes running back, and of course—
they can't stop you. But already I'd found the page, you know. So the
doctor said, "Oh, I forgot the book." He went to take it. I said, "Oh,
what's this on here?" And he, like, looked at me, you know, and he said,
"Oh, that's not important." I said, "It's important to *me!*" I said, "Now,
you're a study hospital." I said, "You're going to take this report," I said,

"saying he's an alcoholic and he smokes and this is what causes cancer." And I said, "Then you wonder why we get upset because the statistics are wrong!"

Jennifer angrily foresees her husband's case being counted as evidence that smoking and alcohol cause cancer. She sees the chart as representing an indictment of her husband's lifestyle and a statement that this lifestyle has caused his illness. Her dialogue with the physician continues:

I said—then I had told him, I said, "That girl thought he was an alcoholic." I said, "She talked to me fifteen minutes," I said, "and diagnosed that from what I said." I said, "She should have asked me how much *did* he drink. She never asked," I said. "And what he was drinking then was," I said, "maybe a case of beer a week." Which comes out to four cans a day. I said, "It's just that the doctor felt the combination might have triggered something off because they couldn't find nothing else." As a matter of fact, he stopped drinking after that. And I said, "I think some of the liquor *kills* these germs in our body if you don't overdo it." And I said, "I drink more than he does. Do I look like an alcoholic?" I was really upset. And he just kept saying to me, "You're concerned about the wrong things."

Jennifer's interest was not solely academic. She wanted the description of her husband as an alcoholic to be taken off his chart.

I said, "I want it off his records." But they never took it off. [MB: They didn't take it off?] No. Then he—then everything was happening too fast, and then I was just tired of arguing with everybody. So—'cause he said, "Oh, I'll have an input put in there." But they never showed it to me.

Jennifer attributes her husband's cancer not to his lifestyle but to his environment. The debate between Jennifer and her husband's physician is the debate between lifestyle and environmental theories of cancer causation.

See, ironically, he got hurt right before this all happened, and I really believed the hurt had caused this. They all said, "No, it doesn't." . . . [MB: He had had like a bad accident or something like that?] Just in work.

Just wrenched his back. Just—and they were treating him for muscle spasm, a muscle pull. . . . He was never sick, until that accident. And then he was wearing a thing around the back and he just kept getting worse and worse and worse. [MB: And it was right after that that he started to lose weight.] This happened in July. By October he was in the hospital.

Jennifer's point is not only that her husband's cancer is connected to his accident but that the power inequity between herself and her husband's physicians caused her observations regarding possible causality to be dismissed. At this point in the interview, I asked her directly about attribution of blame:

[MB: When you were talking about your husband and the doctors, um, I thought that—you know, it was as if they were treating you—that it was his fault somehow? Or you know, that they were saying, "Well, it was because he smoked or because he drank" or something like that, you know?] He didn't actually come out and say that. No, it wasn't said. But when you find out that it's on the report—I'm saying to them, "Let's get *all* the facts together. Not just what you want. I want you to know he did get hurt before this." They didn't want to hear that. You know. "Well, how much does he smoke?" I said, "You know, I'll give you all that information, but take the whole surrounding of what it is! It's not just from the smoking." [MB: I see what you're saying. So it was like they had their ideas and they only wanted the information that filled that in.] 'Cause they're smart. They're smarter than us. They know they are. And they feel this other stuff isn't important, but maybe that's why they aren't getting ahead. [MB: So they never asked those questions—so they don't see that there's a pattern or whatever.] Right. And when I say, "Well, this happened"—they go, "Well, that has nothing to do with it."

Jennifer wanted her husband's chart to include the following information: that he had suffered an accident directly before becoming ill; that he had worked in a chemical plant for many years; and that he lived in a highly polluted neighborhood. She sees these factors as additive, along with lifestyle factors and a measure of fate, in total cancer risk.

Of course, this is a bad neighborhood. He died two years after that explosion, which my neighbor across the street died a year after and they told him it was lung cancer. . . . I really do—I feel it's—now, we all eat the same food at this table. He gets it—I don't. But I think he might have too much in his system. I think we all get it and our system fights it off somehow. Now, when things happen to you—he smoked—which—he got more cancer than I did. He worked at a place that had chemicals so he had more. He lives in a neighborhood that has chemicals. . . . A combination is what I'm telling you. If you probably weigh everything out—I don't think you'll ever beat it. I do believe your time is when it is, too.

Jennifer's challenge left a faint trace on John's medical record. Next to the typewritten words "extensive history of alcohol abuse," there is a marginal notation, handwritten and initialed by the attending physician, that reads: "(less than 1 case of beer/week)."

Death

Upon readmission, John was placed on narcotics for pain relief. He began to have trouble breathing and started to hallucinate. Four days later, a family conference was held, attended by the resident, the attending physician, the social worker, and Jennifer. All agreed that pain control was of primary importance. The resident's note states that Jennifer "is aware of critical nature" and that she requests an autopsy at time of death. The social worker's note states that Jennifer would like to bring John home.

The day after this conference, a morphine drip was started. John began to experience acute respiratory distress, with the type of agitation that accompanies this state. The next day, Haldol, a major tranquilizer, was added to his drip. On that day Jennifer, according to the progress report, became "quite agitated" and wanted to take John home. Hospital staff persuaded her to leave him in the hospital for a few more days, to allow the palliative medications to go into action. The next day's notes read:

[Early a.m.] Wife stayed all nite, as did her sister. Patient-wife are much calmer today. In a.m., plans will be made for homecare.

[9:15 a.m.] No pulse or respiration. Patient expired. No autopsy.

Autopsy

After enduring this long struggle, Jennifer faced one more. She asked that an autopsy be performed. After so much confusion about his diagnosis and anger at the physicians for shutting her out, she felt no sense of resolution at John's death. She reports facing the disapproval of the medical staff:

I had an autopsy done, and they were very upset that I was having the autopsy done, which I was upset—and I said, "Well, I read a few books and they told me this is why youse aren't getting ahead; that enough people aren't autopsying." They felt he had lung cancer. I didn't feel he had lung cancer. I said he never had symptoms. [Hospital D] told me he had stomach cancer. [Hospital F] said, "No, he doesn't. It's lung cancer." I said, "No, it isn't. He never was coughing. He was very athletic. He never got out of breath. He was never spitting up blood." He said to me, "Oh, he had the signs. Youse just didn't look for them." [MB: Well, what was it? I mean, what did the autopsy say?] The pancreas. A different type of cancer. They'd never seen it before. I have the autopsy upstairs. Then I was upset about that after the autopsy. I called the doctor up and he said to me— instead of them telling us—he said to me, "Well, what do you want to know?" I said, "I want to know what you know. I don't know!" He said, "Well, ask me, and I'll tell you." Now, this was at [Hospital F]. And I said, "I don't know what to ask you." I said, "I can read the report, that it was pancreas." I said, "But I just wanted to know everything."
   . . . Well, they don't know anything about it because it's an—they've never seen this type of cancer. That's why the chemo was hard because, uh—the chemo they were giving him was—one type—I don't know what kind. I mean, I have it all upstairs written—but I—like they said to me, "Why do you want an autopsy?" And I said, "I'm not suing." . . . I said, "I just don't feel that's what it was."

Through the autopsy, Jennifer hoped to make sense of her long and troubling struggle regarding medical claims to legitimate knowledge. The question is with her still: did she make the right decisions? The suggestion that it was a difficult case, and the fact that it was misdiagnosed at least twice, provided some explanation, in Jennifer's view, as to why no hospital and no doctor seemed to do well by the patient.[3] But this was small comfort, and the autopsy report lay upstairs, a still-open book at which I was invited to look to help her make sense of the death.

JENNIFER'S VIEW

Jennifer succeeded in finding the best medical care for her husband. Her perceptions that he was receiving suboptimal care at Hospitals B and D were correct. Through challenging medical authority at these institutions and choosing to have John treated at Hospital F, she found state-of-the-art care for him. But even the state of the art had no place for her voice.

Jennifer's ultimate struggle concerned the exclusion of her own voice from her husband's medical record, the authoritative text on his illness and death. Her struggle reached a climax when she challenged the implication that her husband was an alcoholic and that his cancer was attributable to his drinking and smoking. Her challenge was dismissed. She fought this dismissal because it framed her as an observer, and not an actor, in the drama of her husband's death. She also related the dismissal of her views to wider issues concerning medical authority, control, and social class.

The mechanisms of medical dominance are clear in this confrontation. The physician's response to Jennifer—that she is "concerned about the wrong things"—is a veiled moral judgment. It is the same judgment faced by women who resist cesarean sections and voice disappointment at missing the experience of a vaginal delivery (Irwin and Jordan 1987). Medical dominance dictates not only the accepted standard of medical care but the accepted boundaries of patient opinion and emotional response. By the doctrine of personal responsibility for health, patients and their families are culpable if they fail to stay within proscribed behavioral boundaries. When Jennifer does not do so, she is cast as troublesome and described as agitated. As John is judged responsible for his cancer through his poor lifestyle choices, so Jennifer is judged responsible for having illegitimate concerns. Within this framework, however, John's physician is humane and makes a note in the chart. With that note, Jennifer's voice is heard—and placed in the margins. The typed social history, citing alcohol abuse, remains very much the legitimate record. The note beside it is small, handwritten, an afterthought. Despite Jennifer's challenge, John's chart implies that his death was attributable to his lifestyle and that his lifestyle was recklessly unhealthy. Jennifer resists, but her resistance does not become fact in the official statement of her husband's social history. In Scott's terms, domination is not hegemonic, but it remains a social fact (1985:330).

Thus, the power of medical dominance does not determine Jennifer's thoughts and feelings. The "social sphere" in which she speaks freely appears, as Scott says, small only if we view her from within the medical system. This view of Jennifer is radically partial and shuts out her own construction of the events. John's physicians see each confrontation with Jennifer as a moment of trouble in their management of John's case. Jennifer herself constructs these confrontations as moments within her continual struggle to be an effective agent in her own management of the case. With regard first to medical decisions and then to the form of John's final medical record, Jennifer struggles to be included in the dialogue and for her voice to be considered legitimate. Like most people who are the primary support of very sick patients, Jennifer accepts this conflict with medical authority as a major part of her responsibility in caring for John. Although the constraining forces surrounding her are enormous, she persists in being concerned with her own agenda. She accepts the burden of living with the conflict between her own resistance and the social fact of medical dominance. She continues to charge that her voice is being denied.

There are two primary messages that Jennifer wants to document through John's medical record. First, she wants the medical record to say that John's cancer should not be attributed solely to his smoking and drinking. She wants the record to reflect "the whole surrounding of what it is." To Jennifer, John's record states that smoking and alcohol caused his cancer. Shut out of the record, to her eye, are his accident, his industrial exposure, and the fact that he lived in a highly polluted neighborhood. All these factors do appear in the record—as misdiagnosis, name of employer, and address, respectively. But smoking and alcohol take center stage, and occupational and community exposures are not mentioned in any discharge summary or professional correspondence.

In point of fact, alcohol and tobacco use, as factors that have wide and profound impacts on health, should be noted in any medical history. Both are risk factors for pancreatic cancer, and each is relevant to some of the working diagnoses used in John's case (alcohol to gastroenteritis and nonsignificantly to bowel cancer; smoking to both of these and to lung cancer). But alcohol and tobacco are routinely included in medical histories not only because they are relevant to health. They are also lifestyle factors, and therefore they fit the paradigmatic stance in scientific medicine that translates "social history" into a consideration of the ways in which people bear personal responsibility for their health or illness. It is a model that tends to minimize or discount the social, cultural, and environmental contexts of disease. Jennifer's objection speaks directly to this point. She does not object to the inclusion of smoking and alcohol-use history per se. She objects to the exclusion of other factors that she sees as related and to the ease with which the medical staff labels her husband an alcoholic. In both inclusions and exclusions to the medical record, Jennifer sees wider social and political issues at work. In a sense, the basic issue is her right even to enter into a debate about cancer causality. But the factors that she is told have "nothing to do with it" have everything to do with it for her. She fights for their inclusion in the record.

The other message that Jennifer wants included in John's official record is that the physicians who treated him were not infallible and that their claim to a monopoly on legitimacy is unwarranted. Her specific focus here is the issue of diagnosis—an issue on which there was much confusion in John's case, as there often is in cases of pancreatic cancer. At Hospital F, Jennifer challenged the diagnosis of lung cancer. She was aware, as most people are, that medical science sees a strong link between lung cancer and smoking, and she read the diagnosis of lung cancer as a judgment on John. Her challenge to that diagnosis is a challenge to that judgment. When her challenge was rebuffed, she became motivated to order an autopsy. John's physicians denied that her opinions were legitimate; she looked to the autopsy report to deny the legitimacy of *their* opinions. Through the autopsy, she sought to finish a tension, finally to say effectively: *You are not always right, and I am not always wrong; I should have had a voice.*

In one sense, the autopsy bolsters Jennifer in this feeling, by establishing that the primary site of John's cancer was not the lung, but the pancreas. Hospital F physicians had considered pancreatic cancer as a possible working diagnosis, and complications from metastases to the lungs were the proximal cause of John's death. But to Jennifer, the misdiagnosis demonstrates that it was illegitimate for the physicians to shut her out and blame John for his disease. She was not at the time aware that smoking is also a risk factor for pancreatic cancer—nor does this now make a difference in her reading of the social process behind John's diagnosis. In another sense, however, the autopsy only provided another occasion for Jennifer to be rebuffed. Years later, one of Jennifer's clearest memories is the refrain of the pathologist: "Well, what do you want to know?" To the end, and beyond, her sense of defiance is both bolstered and dismissed. She is left with an enduring conflict.

At root, what Jennifer sought to challenge was the medical profession's control of the meaning of her husband's death. Despite her efforts, his life slipped from her grasp. Then, the final medical judgment on his life remained beyond her control, as well. Expropriating the meaning of his death, medical science expropriated her ability to feel closure, to experience herself as having been an agent for good in her husband's life, and to construct their life together as having been a worthy one and not the cause of his death. In the physician's eyes, the medical record is objective. To Jennifer, it privileges an apolitical frame for a political statement. John's medical record denies politically sensitive assertions about cancer causation, refuses to acknowledge her analysis of medicine as a social system, and constructs her as an agitated wife. Jennifer steadfastly stuck to her interpretations, but this was not without its costs. The autopsy did not bring closure—it served to bring the conflict into clearer focus. Years later, she is unable to put this conflict to rest.

After John's death, Jennifer continued to live in Tannerstown. A few years later, her father died, leaving his bar to her. Although she knew nothing about running a bar, she decided to try to make a go of it. She and her mother traded domiciles, her mother moving back to the Tannerstown house, and Jennifer and her three children moving to the apartment above the bar. To her great delight, she has made a success of the business, and it has renewed her sense of control over her life. But she has not put John's death to rest and still seeks to legitimize her claim that he was not to blame for his cancer. Her agreement to work with me speaks to her continuing effort. Ironically, now that her insights are written in a book, they gain some measure of legitimacy. Her voice is finally, in a sense, added to the medical record.

THE PHYSICIAN'S VIEW

Up to this point in my description of John's case, Jennifer is the only character I have drawn clearly. She is represented by her own voice, which is vivid and intelligent. In contrast, the physicians involved are represented indirectly, by Jennifer's recollections and by the text of John's medical record.

So often, this is the case in medical anthropology. Patients and their families, and lay people in general, are often more accessible, and perhaps less intimidating, to anthropologists—most of whom prefer, in any case, to listen to the voices of the less powerful.

This preference can simplify our view of the medical encounter. It is easy to connect lay critiques of medicine to wider conceptual frameworks dealing with power, politics, economics, and conflict and to trace the labyrinthine manifestations of medical authority through various contexts and cases. Such an analysis can stand, *quod erat demonstrandum,* as an analysis of medicine as a social system. But in such a rendering, both patients and physicians appear only as caricatures. The patient is a hapless victim, and the physician is an embodiment of all-powerful forces. The medical encounter is a series of crude power moves, in which the physician wields a sledgehammer, and the patient cringes or fights back.

In Jennifer's story, we see nothing of the physician's consciousness of Jennifer's challenge to medical authority or of the physician's experience of his or her own power in the climactic confrontation with Jennifer. Nor should we expect to. To begin to understand the physician's experience, we must turn to the physician.

A number of years after John's death, I was able, using information from his medical record from Hospital F, to locate one of the attending physicians on his case. This physician graciously agreed to an interview. I originally wrote the section that follows without giving this physician a name: I realized on a later draft that this was refusing him the humanity that I had automatically thought to assign to John and Jennifer. I have therefore assigned him the pseudonym Dr. Hughes.

When I described John's case to Dr. Hughes, he remembered John but did not remember the confrontation with Jennifer or any details about John's social history. After a brief discussion of the case, I presented Jennifer's critique to Dr. Hughes, point by point. I began with Jennifer's assertion that physicians put in the medical record only that which affirms the views they already hold. The tape recorder begins a few words into Dr. Hughes's answer:

So I think it is true that—that most physicians look for what they—you know, want to expect. And ninety-nine percent of the time we're probably correct in making those assumptions, uh—in this instance, somebody saying that they drink, or a—a family member recounting that a patient drinks a—a—case of beer a week, generally speaking people underreport alcohol intake, and then there are studies to show that. And usually by a factor of two. That is, one-half to two-thirds. So, if somebody is saying they're drinking a, uh, case of beer a week, it's probably two and three cases a week. And that's a lot of beer. . . . As far as, uh, doctors including the work history and exposure history and the environment, I would think most doctors don't because they're not educated in that area; very few doctors have had sufficient epidemiology training to—or public health training—to look or even question that. Unless the patient would bring it out and would talk about some pretty gross exposure. But, ah—or unless a diagnosis would come forward that would s—for instance, uh, a neurologic problem that might lead to a suspicion of lead—intoxication which might then lead to very specific questions about working with batteries or working with, uh, lining, uh, uh, you know, brake linings and things like that. So unless one got, you know, some hints from the workup of the patient, we probably don't do a very adequate—environmental—uh, history.

Dr. Hughes accedes to Jennifer's criticism. Yes, he says, we do include the details we most expect to hear. He defends the expert authority of the physician: we are, he says, usually on the right track; and it is known through studies that patients tend to underreport alcohol use. But his defense is not emotional, and with regard to the slighting of environmental factors in medical histories, he simply agrees with Jennifer's point. Although he contradicts some of what Jennifer says, Dr. Hughes is not tied to or motivated by a need to prove her definitively wrong point by point. His tone toward me is patient and not at all defensive. He seems accustomed to admitting his failings and the failings of his profession.

Again, I asked Dr. Hughes about his confrontation with Jennifer. The physician's emotions are often complex, he answered, and each case is different. But then he spoke of the psychosocial issue that would have been, in his view, important for most oncologists in such a confrontation. In the following passage, he offers his interpretation:

You have to re—understand that, yeah, there are frequently confrontations like this. Where, ah, here you can give the person your advice, you can tell them that this is important . . . and, ah, yet she doesn't want to listen to that at all . . . I—I think what—what people, what—what physicians learn in their training, and what they by nature begin to do, is become authoritarian to a certain extent, I mean, you have to tell people rather positively— you *must* take this medicine and you *must* do this and, ah, you know, because this is what's *best* for you. Well, patients, in this modern age interpret that as being—you know, not having their own—authority, not having their own—being in control of their own destiny. And so there's *always* this kind of push and pull between people who, ah, who wanna be in control and those physicians who are trying to outline the best *treatment* for the patient. [MB: Do you think that—that those issues are, um, ah—really especially central in oncology?] Well, maybe more so, ah—obviously it's more serious 'cause a mistake is usually a—a—life threatening, you know, or *fatal* mistake. In fact if you *don't* do the right thing up front that's usually where the fa-fatalities occur. So, ah—[MB: You mean if the—if the *physician* doesn't do the right thing.] Yeah, and the—and the patient. See, if the patient delays, or decides that he—he wants to continue to seek opinions until he finds an opinion that coincides with *his* desires, that may be in fact a *fatal* mistake for him. [MB: Uh-huh. Wow.] So, ah, so, oncologists

probably more than most specialists have to become much more, um—
[MB: Forceful.] controlling. [MB: Clear, and—] Yeah. And—and—and,
uh—and we frequently hear that, you know, nobody di-discussed this
with—well, I *pretty* well—I know a *lot* of oncologists, and they usually go
out of their way to explain what's going on, and we usually don't use
euphemisms like, ah, this could be a tumor or this could be a little lump.
We usually talk, it's cancer and you've got to do this, and—and yet patients
still seem to not hear what the doctor is saying.

To Dr. Hughes, the issue is not that the physician is too controlling, it
is that the physician cannot control enough. He understands the needs
of patients "in this modern age" to feel in control but sees this need as
an adversary, "push and pull," to his own control of the treatment
decision at stake. If the physician fails to control that treatment decision, the result is loss of life. Dr. Hughes stumbles over the word
"fatalities," and puts heavy stress on the word "fatal," which is spoken
twice. He stresses the idea that fatal mistakes are made in the beginning. Thus, he assumes an extraordinary burden: that of insuring that
both physician and patient make the right decisions, at a time when
the consequences of those decisions are not yet clear.

   To Dr. Hughes, it is this consciousness of mortality that causes the
physician to become "authoritarian." Where I choose "forceful," a
kinder word, he insists on "controlling." And yet what strikes him, in
the end, is that the physician is in the final analysis unable to control—
partly, in his eyes, through being unable to communicate clearly
enough with patients and their families.

   My interview with Dr. Hughes then moved to a discussion of Jennifer's position. I opened the topic by describing Jennifer's frustration in
trying to make the right decisions about John's care. Dr. Hughes cut
into my description, the only instance in the interview in which he
directly and aggressively interrupted me:

[MB: And she did in fact make a lot of decisions and good ones.] But
[MB: I mean, after all—] But why—why *should* she be the one making
them? [MB: Um—] You see, I think she's assuming a lot of things that
aren't—[MB: Yeah?] [*Pause*] Generally speaking, we feel the patient should
make the decisions. Now, obviously family members should be present and

should *hear* the information, but usually I—tend to reject—a family member—making the decisions for the patient. Because, ah, after all, it is still the patient that has to go *through* the treatment, or has to bear the results of, uh, of whatever the problem is. So in a sense, ah, that's very presumptuous on her part, that she should be telling her husband what— should happen, or telling the doctors how to treat her husband. [MB: Right. And of course I have no—*no* way of knowing anything, about the patient. I mean, there's a social worker's note here and there about things that he had said, but—] But I'm sure he was very reticent, and very quiet, and probably withdrawn, and—maybe depressed. And, ah, you know, in—in pediatrics it's—it's usual for the mother to answer for the child. And—and, you know, and decision making. But in adults, we generally reject that.

With some vehemence, Dr. Hughes insists that his moral responsibility and primary relationship is to the patient. He presents this as a central tenet of medical practice. Still, this passage must be read in the context of Dr. Hughes's earlier descriptions of the patient-physician relationship as fraught with oppositions and endangered by struggles for control. In rejecting family authority over the patient, the physician experiences a construction of himself as tied to the patient by bonds of common interest. The family is cast as among the many threats to physician control, as being outsiders to the primary patient-physician tie. Again, Dr. Hughes returns to the central nightmare of physician loss of control:

It's a very complex specialty, it's one that takes, ah, a lot of time but also a lot of detail, ah, applied, eh, small errors or mistakes, uh, frequently are fatal. [*Pause*] They—they don't *appear* to be, right at that moment, but— but they probably add up to be—fatal for the patient, ah, in a short time, or long time.

The beginning of this passage is spoken slowly, word by word, until the words "frequently are fatal." This phrase is spoken in a rush, as one word, with a short pause following. In oncology practice, death is a constant companion. For Dr. Hughes, it is the only important foe. It is, to paraphrase his admonition to Jennifer, the right thing to be concerned about.

In medical oncology, more so than in some other areas of medicine, the concerns of families are an enormous emotional burden, one that is sometimes beyond bearing for the already emotionally exhausted physician. In a way, families and physicians may suffer from the same emotional burden: anger about the patient's cancer. This may be especially so in a case with a poor prognosis. But this anger, if it does indeed animate confrontations such as that between Jennifer and Dr. Hughes, is not felt as a commonality. Adversarial understandings of the medical encounter structure the interpretations of all participants and suggest a target of anger for each. Through such understandings, oncologists and patient's families may often be pitted against each other, in a complex of angry emotions that everyone is too overwhelmed to sort out.

Common angers notwithstanding, Jennifer and Dr. Hughes brought different issues to their confrontation with each other. Jennifer did not want John blamed for his cancer. Because this is her interpretation of the conflict between herself and the physician, she attributed to the physician the point of view that John should be blamed. But Jennifer and Dr. Hughes confront each other at cross-purposes. Dr. Hughes understands that medical records recreate and reaffirm the expectations of physicians, and he sees that this process can reify the view that cancer is caused by patient lifestyles. But to Dr. Hughes, this is not the important issue. It is not what he is defensive about, or the answer he ultimately comes to, or his interpretation of why he pushed Jennifer away. His central concern is in maintaining control, because to lose control is to be responsible for his patient's death.

In earlier chapters, I described my experiences in the Tannerstown community and detailed local views on cancer causation, social class, and medical authority. In this chapter, I have presented a case study involving the cancer death of a Tannerstown resident. Two important questions arise. First, what practical lessons might clinicians and patients draw from John's case history? Second, how are the clinical and community contexts related? In developing answers to these questions, I will offer three separate readings of John's case.

My first reading highlights the commonality between my story of the community and my story of the clinic. The commonality is clear. In both community and clinic, Tannerstowners voice a resistance to professional authorities that would blame them, openly or tacitly, for their cancer. John's case, and the confrontation between Jennifer and Dr. Hughes, may be read as a bit of lived, felt experience that illustrates the specific workings of wider social forces such as medical authority and class discrimination.

When they confront each other, Jennifer and Dr. Hughes both seek to forge a concrete response to the wider fields of power in which they are enmeshed and must act. In both of them, one sees the pain of people who are trying to do what they think is right and important, and to act concretely to defend what they value. Jennifer's struggle is about meaning and the official documentation of truth. To the confrontation with Dr. Hughes, she brings long experience that has taught her that people like her do not participate in the construction of truth. Now, she seeks to be a writer of truth, a writer of the story of her own husband's death. For his part, Dr. Hughes struggles to be an effective physician. His definition of effective action is narrowly constrained by his professional training and what it has taught him: a focus on the patient's body, a focus on life as in danger, a focus on his own responsibility to that body and that life, a focus on staying focused at all costs. Dr. Hughes defends himself against the undoing of focus that Jennifer demands of him. In the final analysis, of course, he holds more power than she does. His voice is recorded as real, and hers is not.

Virtually all patients experience such differences in power between themselves and their physicians. Our picture of life in Tannerstown, Jennifer and John's community, however, suggests that the issues of cancer causation and social-class power differences were linked for Jennifer prior to her confrontation with Dr. Hughes. Jennifer's strong sense of the issue of relative power is colored by the depth of this prior link. Interestingly, Jennifer does not talk explicitly about social class. Her dominant metaphors for social class are education and intelligence. She speaks of the physicians at Hospital F as being "too smart" and as "smarter than us." Thus, on both semantic and strategic levels, she casts a social-class struggle as a struggle about intelligence, knowledge, and truth. In one interview, she phrased it as follows:

> I was never good at asking questions the right way, or expressing myself the right way. And people like that—I guess we'll have a hard time, when you're in the medical field, if they're not with the right doctor that's going to sit down and say, "I know you don't understand, let's go over this." . . . Why do they treat them so different? An educated person comes in there, they *do* treat them different. . . . And it's a way of telling us, "Well, you're not smart enough to understand this." And I did feel that a lot, you know. And, uh, "I shouldn't be wasting my time cause you wouldn't understand it anyway." Yeah, I felt that way a lot.

"People like that" are people who are labeled in school as not intelligent; who are told that they cannot understand things as well; who have less formal education; who are told they are "not smart enough." In this language, we see the insidious and destructive confounding of school success and intelligence that is so common in our society. "People like that" clearly refers to Tannerstowners, or to working-class people in general. Elsewhere in that same interview, I asked Jennifer directly about social class. She drew a blank. She speaks of social class only in terms of a self-deprecating mystification.

What Dr. Hughes brings to the meeting, with respect to wider social forces that shape the interaction, is not class discrimination but medical authority. In this, Dr. Hughes serves as an interesting example. My judgment of Dr. Hughes is that he is not particularly prone to social-class prejudice. In fact, I read him as a person who freely enjoys fraternal relationships with people of various social backgrounds. In my few observations of him with patients, he appeared very open to their suggestions and not defensive about their critiques. But in this first reading of the case, that is beside the point. Dr. Hughes still represents those who are hated for their class power, and he is still committed to authority as a keystone of effective medical practice.

My first reading, then, illustrates themes already discussed in my examination of the social dynamics between Tannerstown and Project CAN-DO. The force of collision between Tannerstown and the cancer science establishment—on a wider level, between the working class and the medical establishment—reverberates within the specific meeting between Jennifer and Dr. Hughes. Such a reading springs from a stance common in critical medical anthropology, in which prior insight into wider political and economic structures of power order perceptions of individual interactions. Such a stance orders the world very strongly and gives the analyst a firm commitment. This appeals to many academics in the United States, where we are fond of conceptual order, are comfortable with absolute heroes and villains, and are currently feeling bereft of a stable place from which to analyze. Thus, Jennifer is our hero, and Dr. Hughes, with perhaps some sympathetic caveats, is our villain. John's case, as noted above, is illustration and brightens up the narrative with a human-interest story. Human experience in the service of conceptual structure: this is indeed an alienated use of lived experience. It also offers us no practical suggestions and only a mechanistic tie between clinic and community.

My second reading of John's case will take us somewhat further. This second reading will be from the perspective of clinical medical anthropology, as defined by the work of Arthur Kleinman (Kleinman 1980, 1981; Kleinman, Eisenberg, and Good 1978). This reading will focus strongly on cognition within the clinic.

Kleinman's perspective—that of a physician-anthropologist widely respected in both anthropology and medicine—is that scientific medicine has great powers to make people well and that the improvement of patient compliance is a good goal for anthropologists who study the clinic. At the center of Kleinman's view is the concept of Explanatory Models (EMs)—that is, the cultural constructs of clinical reality that both patient and physician bring to the clinical encounter. This focus highlights cognitive disparities between patient and physician and defines communication as the basic problem. Kleinman argues for more culturally sensitive clinical practice. He distinguishes between disease (a physical phenomenon) and illness (a cultural phenomenon), like many medical anthropologists, and he exhorts anthropologists to teach physicians to treat both. This microsociological focus is strategic and programmatic, privileging a microsociological outcome: patient compliance.

Kleinman tells us that "generally speaking, the explanatory models of professional practitioners are oriented toward disease while those of the laity are oriented toward illness" (1980:73). This is certainly an accurate reading of the dissonance between Jennifer and Dr. Hughes. Jennifer openly insists on the relevance of social context and is concerned with the social construction of definitions, whereas Dr. Hughes insists on a concern with physical disease. Kleinman's model points us in the direction of these relatively opaque cognitions and suggests that if Jennifer and Dr. Hughes had negotiated an effective communication about what was important to each of them, Jennifer would not be left with so much unresolved emotional pain. This perspective has merit. If Dr. Hughes had stated that environment could have played a role in John's cancer—if he had, for instance, made the simple assertion that cancer causation is complex and physicians are often not sure how it develops in any given patient—it might have reduced Jennifer's suffering. Jennifer herself seems to believe this. Throughout, she represents herself as searching for communication. For instance, at one point, she changes hospitals in a search for a physician who can communicate better with her. At another point, she regrets that she never had an interview with the pathologist and seems to feel that in such a communication, she might have found what she wanted.

Thus, Kleinman offers an answer for one of our questions—that is, what concrete recommendations we might propose for reform of the clinic. Within the confines of the clinic, Kleinman's answer is a good one. With regard to our second question, however—that is, how to tie analyses of the clinic to analyses of wider social contexts—this answer needs amendment.

Kleinman considers the wider context, and states his wider ideal as follows:

Anthropological medicine and psychiatry would seek to alter the power relationships within the health care system such that care became more patient-centered and the practitioner-patient relationship approximated a *negotiation* between relative equals in which the practitioner provided expert information, but the patient and family retained the responsibility for accepting or rejecting such advice. Again, this change would require preceding external alterations in power relationships in order to be effected. (Kleinman 1981:171; emphasis in the original)

But whether they negotiate a shared EM or not, Jennifer and Dr. Hughes will never meet as equals. As Kleinman acknowledges in this passage, deep change within the clinic needs change outside the clinic. Nothing Dr. Hughes does can change Jennifer's lifelong experiences. He cannot, through better communication, alter the fact of the chemical plant explosion in Tannerstown, which plays a significant role in Jennifer's EM about John's cancer. We cannot move in a linear fashion from a clinical perspective to the wider world. As critical medical anthropology can cause us to miss the specificity of the clinical encounter, so clinical medical anthropology does not provide a conceptual basis, pure and simple, for apprehending social reality outside the clinic, or for connecting clinical reality to wider contexts. This is recognized by many critical and clinical anthropologists, including Kleinman himself.

Community and clinic cannot be tied together in a simple way— either by using the clinic as illustration, or by formulating our goals within the clinic. Lessons, models, and perspectives from one context do not suffice for viewing the other. The analytical edifices we construct as academics are too transcendent, permanent, and consistent, and too rational and lucid across contexts, to fit real life. In the story I tell here, however, there is a thematic consonance between clinic and community—a consonance that neither of the above two readings can catch. What is missing is a recognition of emotion. In the case study, emotion shows us politics and social context as they are experienced on a personal scale. Emotion and cognition are not opposed: as Michelle Rosaldo says, "feeling is forever given shape through thought and . . . thought is laden with emotional meaning" (1984:143). Still, without tracing emotion, we miss seeing how social class and medical authority are embodied in individual lives (compare Rosaldo 1984). In the present case history, in which cancer, social class, and medical authority are tied together with fear, anger, and moral passion, emotion illuminates a lot. Emotion, then, will be the focus of my third reading.

One key moment of dramatic emotion in Jennifer's story centers on her insistence that John's medical record not define him as an alcoholic. At this moment, she confronts Dr. Hughes and demands that

John's drinking habits be fairly described. During one of our interviews, when Jennifer and I reviewed John's hospital record together, she saw Dr. Hughes's notation "less than 1 case of beer/week" for the first time. When she saw it, she leaned forward intently and I saw worry and effort flood her face.

[MB: Okay, page twenty-seven, it says "less than 1 case of beer per week." So, remember when you said, "I want that written down on the chart"?] That's where he added it? Where does it say—also, "there's a twenty-two-year history—" Here, now, where does it say there that—ah, for drinking, in here—[MB: It says—this is "SH," social history, so—] Oh! [MB: "Patient is married, fairly extensive history of alcohol abuse—" See, they're repeating the same thing.] Yeah. . . . I remember Dr. Hughes rushing in so fast cause he had to go on to his next meeting, wherever he was going, and somehow by instinct I felt, they're looking at me like, "well, you have nothing else to complain about. I know you're upset about him dying, so you're just picking on us." But it was my true feeling. My true feeling was, it wasn't true. If you're ever going to do anything, do the research right. . . . It didn't look like much of a big deal to them. Which I see it wasn't a big deal. They didn't even give it a paragraph. [MB: Right. Like a pinprick. It's not typed or anything.] Right, right, they just gave it a little—which I'm even surprised they did that. I always wondered if it was written in there. But let someone taste a beer—! It's almost exactly what I said, but that isn't correct. That didn't correct anything that I wanted it to correct.

Her words are included in the medical record—but the words do not correct anything. The words do not speak to her "true feeling," which was that John was not to blame for his cancer. They blame him, she says, for just tasting a beer—the smallest transgression, and they blame the patient. There is no emotional closure, no closure in spirit, from the fact that her few words were written in the margin. That does not correct the feelings she is left with.

Another powerful moment of emotion is Jennifer's description of the rudeness of the pathologist. In this moment, the pathologist resists talking to Jennifer about the autopsy. Jennifer has referred to this every time she has told me her story. It clearly continues to haunt her.

I was just very disappointed that I didn't have an interview. He called and said he was busy, he can answer me on the phone. . . . "Well, what do you want to know?" I didn't know. I said, "What *you* know." And he said, "Well, it took me years to go to school and I couldn't tell you that." That hurt.

Again, the injury is emotional, and so is the closure she needs. From the written autopsy report, she has what she wants to *know:* that she was right, John's primary disease was not lung cancer. This reads to her as a factual statement that he is not to blame for his disease. What she does not have is what she wants to *feel,* which is a sense of effectiveness as an agent for her husband, in his life and in his death. The rational fact in the autopsy does not provide that.

I would draw a third example from my interview with Dr. Hughes. The most emotional moment in this interview is when Dr. Hughes expresses the primacy of his own private relationship with his patient. When I say that Jennifer had made good decisions, he interrupts and asks, with emotional heat, "why *should* she be the one making them?" He expresses the view that his primary responsibility as John's physician is to communicate directly with John. He frames this as an ethical issue, tying his emotional vehemence to a "should." The stance he takes, however, is not a timeless ethical stance. Professional mores about open talk to cancer patients have changed through time in the United States, toward more open, direct communication with patients, and still differ from country to country, even within the realm of scientific medicine. But clearly, for Dr. Hughes, emotion and ethical sense are tied, perhaps specifically with the energy of anger; and deeply felt emotions are confounded with ideals to which he holds himself with regard to caring for and about his patients.

At first, this emotion-centered reading of John's case seems unconnected to my first reading, which was concerned with power and wider social forces. The focus on emotion, however, speaks to a central paradox in my first reading: how John's case can be about class and authority, and refer to class and authority, in cognitive and rational terms, so thinly. Emotion is the tie. The emotions expressed by both Jennifer and Dr. Hughes are the specific costs to them of life in the context of wider forces. Neither of them experiences social class and medical authority as such, and these rational structural edifices are not written into the case history verbatim. But many of the emotions they feel *are* class and authority in the form of lived experience. Disputes about class and authority are etched into their lives with pain, depression, exhaustion, anger, and all the rest. They are both transformed in the process.

The third reading also extends the second, by drawing us away from the confines of cognition and EMs. Medical authority is too big to fit into an EM. When we make it fit, we strip it of visible signs of its purpose. Doctor Hughes's EM, for instance, even if reformed as per Kleinman's suggestions, would still be rooted in a complex hope for patient compliance, because therein lies the best hope of cure. Likewise, working-class experience—in this case, growing up and living in Tannerstown—is too big to fit into an EM. When we make it fit, we strip it of the holistic perceptions and experiences of working-class people. Jennifer, for instance, still thinks about Tannerstown and still broods about whether air and water pollution pose health risks for her children. When rich and complex life processes are poured into EMs, they are reconstructed in the process and cleansed for the specific job at hand. "Medical authority" and "social class" become "barriers to communication." Again, this constitutes an alienated use of lived experience. The root problem in the clinic is not a problem of communication. It is a problem of power.

In the end, all three readings of John's case are best taken together. As suggested in the first reading, we see in the clinic what we saw in the community: working-class life experience and the workings of medical authority. As suggested by the second, failures of communication in the clinic are great cruelties, and we can stand in favor of Kleinman's suggestions for reform. But the third reading adds a sensibility through which we can make sense of community and clinic as a whole. In John's case, medical authority is sometimes muddled, and we are barely able to catch a glimpse of social class. Instead, we see the pain of unresolvable emotions. This speaks not to the weakness of class images but to the powerful and subtle forms through which they come into play.

MEANING FOR THE ANTHROPOLOGIST $\Big|5\Big|$

It is in moments of crisis, when the routines of ordinary life are held in abeyance, that people most dramatically bring into focus and negotiate a sense of meaning for their lives.

Michael Jackson and Ivan Karp, Introduction to *Personhood and Agency*

And although one might be excused for occasionally doubting it—for such is professional rhetoric—anthropologists are social beings too.

Michael Herzfeld, *Anthropology through the Looking-glass*

As people in Europe and the United States have had their perceptions of world dominance shaken and transformed, anthropologists have come to appreciate the politics and historicity of the views we take of the Other.[1] In *Anthropology through the Looking-glass,* Michael Herzfeld offers a particularly disturbing challenge to the traditional anthropological stance. He asserts that the constructions of the world that we invent as professional anthropologists are the forms through which we muse about our own experience. The structures, oppositions, dilemmas, and enduring conflicts that we read as the "culture" of the people we study reflect and are reflections of our own preoccupations with and for our own lives.

In my story so far, I have looked at Tannerstowners, health educators, a patient's wife, and an oncologist and have traced their efforts to negotiate the burdens and powers of medical authority. The next character I will look at is the applied anthropologist in the story— that is, myself. Following Herzfeld's admonition, I will attempt to treat my own conceptual edifices about the world around me and about my struggle to define a sense of meaning for my life as material for social analysis, rather than as a privileged analytical mode of thought. To that end, I will return to my critique of health education.

At the time of my employment at Fox Chase, this critique was a keystone in my own sense of moral legitimacy, both personal and professional. I will reread my critique of health education as a reaction to my own personal dilemmas. By doing so, I hope to further my wider discussion of social-class conflict and the burdens of professional authority, and my description of the ways in which these edifices are experienced.

HEALTH EDUCATOR AS "OTHER"

My critique of health education was developed not in a vacuum but in the context of my professional position at Fox Chase. In many ways, my position was painful. I had first been hired at Fox Chase as a health educator, in a Master's-level position. I was soon dismayed to learn that my Ph.D., in this doctoral-rich medical environment, meant next to nothing. For the first two weeks of my employment, I kept waiting to be taken to the office of the vice-president for cancer control, to be introduced as the new colleague on board. It never happened. A month or so after I was hired, I was with another health educator, walking through the lunch room in the main building at the center. We crossed paths with the vice-president, and my colleague introduced us. The vice-president was pleasant and welcoming. I was hit by a realization that I was unimportant within the organization.

My supervisor—the principal investigator and director of Project CAN-DO—rode out my frustrations and continued to put in front of me the idea that I should begin my ethnographic study. But as I became more acquainted with the health-education setting and became accepted both at work and in the community as a health educator, I began to invest in the effort to be a good one. As I did so, I experienced a split perception. On one hand, I feared being incompetent in this foreign field. On the other hand, I developed what I perceived as an analytical distance from it, by developing a critique of health-education practice.

I have stated my critique of health education in preceding chapters but will briefly restate it here. I see health education as a field caught between two powerful forces. On one side is scientific medicine; on the other, a community or patient population defined as needing education, generally because of some form of noncompliance. The social and instrumental dominance of physicians in the health field, including granting agencies, pushes health educators into the role of handmaid to the medical establishment. This rebounds into the culture of health education and depoliticizes it in ways that scientific medicine requires. Health education is therefore committed to medicalization and to other forms of judgment against the nonadherent. The central morality of health education, however, is one of service to and respect for community or patient. Health educators are often motivated by a morality of social activism and advocacy for the lay public. This is not promoted by medical dominance. Thus, this dominance brings about distortions in professional practice that are often painfully felt by health educators—and pointed to caustically by the lay people with whom they work. It is hard for health educators to escape medical dominance. The field needs to be politicized, gain independence, confront issues like industrial pollution and cancer, and listen to community critiques. The residents of Tannerstown want to escape from the authority of scientific medicine—health educators must learn to want the same thing.

This perspective is well established in the field of health promotion, and has been powerfully expressed by others.[2] Still, in my own experience, it sprang fully formed from my own head, before I developed any familiarity with the literature in health promotion. My critique was not based on a depth of understanding rooted in years of experience. There was an automatic, inescapable quality to it, and I held it with an enormous sense of emotional commitment.

What interests me here is the way in which this critique functioned for me, as a statement about conflicts I felt in my own professional identity at Fox Chase. I contend that my critique came so easily because it was based on a deep imperative, rooted in my own struggle for professional self-definition, to cast health educators as Other to my Self as an applied anthropologist.

APPLIED ANTHROPOLOGIST AS "SELF"

In my construction of health educators as Other, my purpose was to construct a morally superior vantage point for myself. My critique of health educators said that as an anthropologist, I was not a handmaid; I was not apolitical; I was able to see clearly; I did not in the final analysis fail to advocate for or listen to the community I championed.

This stance on the part of anthropologists, but particularly, I think, applied anthropologists, is fairly common. Some of our finest and most impressive case studies—I am thinking of the Washington Area Practicing Anthropologists Praxis Award winners (see Wulff and Fiske 1987)—take a self-congratulatory, often slightly amused tone toward those whose investigations lack "the anthropological difference." Certainly, applied anthropologists have a lot to be proud of, but there is professional insecurity, even defensiveness, between the lines.

Like health education, applied anthropology is an enterprise beset by conflicts. The critiques we develop of other professions are shaped, in part, as a response to conflicts in our own field. This is exemplified by and reflected in my own situation. I will examine this by describing three important conflicts in applied anthropology, and for each, detail the ways in which my critique of health education served to mitigate these conflicts for me.

The first conflict for applied anthropologists involves the yearning to be seen as professionally competent. Most people share this yearning, but applied anthropologists experience it under difficult circumstances. Applied anthropologists are often called upon to develop professional competence within other fields—often fields that are defined as more technical, or more scientific, than our home discipline. Within the hierarchy of academic prestige in the United States, possessing technical and scientific skills encourages a certain type of smugness. Applied anthropologists can feel even more superior than that: we can meet the scientifically competent on their own ground, but we also possess the anthropological difference. It takes energy to maintain such feelings of competence—in a world dominated by quantitative methodologies, anthropologists are often suspect. Recasting other professionals with whom we work as "natives" is one way of defending against this challenge. We resist being judged by setting ourselves up as judges.

My own experience serves as an example. At Fox Chase, I did yearn to be seen as competent. I put energy into familiarizing myself with the basic literature in health education and with some of the social-psychology theory that informs practice in that field. I tried to absorb as much medical knowledge about cancer as I could. I felt that I had not only to prove myself as a health educator but also to prove the usefulness of anthropology. Powerful colleagues from other fields dictated the expenditure of my professional energies, and I responded with a drive to succeed according to their dictates. It was difficult. I sometimes felt that I had to choose between becoming competent in their field and staying competent in my own. In this context, my critique of health education enabled me to feel that I did indeed have a competent view of their field. This view was my own, in some part a secret. It was an anthropological analysis. Through it, I felt that I had a competent grasp of my own professional world.

A second common conflict for applied anthropologists is engendered when our own codes of professional ethics differ from those of colleagues in other fields. I am not talking about specifics regarding such matters as informant confidentiality—such issues can be complex, but at least we have clear general principles to guide us. I am speaking of conflicts that threaten our general sense that we are leading an ethical professional life. Different fields have different sensibilities in this regard. Because of the history of our field, anthropologists are obsessed with the ethical dangers of assuming authority over other people. But this obsession runs counter to the medicalization that is at the heart of the health-education enterprise. For instance, for the health educators with whom I worked, changing peoples' behavior was an ethical goal. This goal made me uncomfortable. I saw elements in it of the desire to improve peoples' lives. I also saw an assumption of authority I did not like. Again, my critique of health education mitigated my felt conflict. If, as Clifford (1986) suggests, ethnography and theory can be read as allegory, my critique of health education can be read as an allegory through which, representing myself to myself, I told myself that I was the only true advocate for the community—the only one who truly listened, the only one who truly understood. I was therefore refusing to assume an authority that I did not believe to be ethical. This allegory, as self-representation, was dear to me—as it is for many anthropologists. It was *my* way to claim an ethical stance.

A third common conflict for applied anthropologists, closely related to the first two but worthy of separate mention, is tied to our habit of defining ourselves as separate from the worlds in which we live. In some subtle way, holding ourselves analytically apart supports our feeling of moral defensibility. When we define ourselves as observers everywhere, we feel our practice is moral. But the cost of this is conflicts about professional loyalties that never really get solved. In my own case, when I was employed at Fox Chase, I was conflicted about who my audience was. As a health educator speaking to other health educators, I would have been happy with the idea that I was understanding community worldviews well enough to design more effective programs. For health educators, this is defined as culturally sensitive practice. But what is this an allegory for? This stance, taken as an allegory, says that health educators strengthen their claim to rightful authority over others when they better understand other cultures. Obviously, this is not a professional stance to which an anthropologist can easily feel loyal. It assumes a crude concept of culture. It also constitutes a use of ethnographic authority to augment the authority of health promotion. Holding myself analytically apart did nothing to help me with this conflict.

These three conflicts beset applied anthropologists when they are working in the "applied world." In applied work, anthropologists usually work in close association with colleagues from other fields. What is more, these colleagues are often more powerful than the anthropologist. As my own experience illustrates, our critiques of the professions of Others are constructed in part to defend our Selves from our own professional insecurities.

There is a fourth central conflict to consider, one that was central to my own feelings of discomfort in my professional life at Fox Chase. This fourth conflict is central not only for applied anthropologists but for other anthropologists as well. It animates a division within the discipline and springs from conflicts at the heart of the anthropological stance. To introduce a discussion of this last and very powerful conflict, I will resume my personal narrative and describe my own turn to the academic world.

CONFLICT IN THE ACADEMY

I worked as a health educator on Project CAN-DO for about a year and a half. At the end of that time, my ethnographic study was well under way, and I had read a well-received paper at a national meeting of cancer-control researchers. The principal investigator of Project CAN-DO had just announced that she was leaving her post at Fox Chase and had made clear to the vice-president that he should consider inviting me to become an investigator. As I understood it, there had been some talk of my being given the opportunity to write my own grant proposal. I constructed an elaboration of the ethnographic project I had begun, which would fit with the continuation of Project CAN-DO. At the principal investigator's urging, I made an appointment with the vice-president to discuss my research interests.

At this time, the Cancer Control Division was facing a serious funding challenge. In less than three months the proposal for renewal of our National Cancer Institute program project grant was due. Program project grants fund a core infrastructure to support research—statistical and computer support staff, secretarial and clerical assistance, and a small percentage of the time of key long-range planners—plus at least three research projects. An applicant—generally a large institution—could propose more than three research projects, and more than three could be approved; but if at least three were not fundable on their own merits, the entire program project grant proposal would be denied.

I was not in sufficient touch with power knowledge networks to understand my own position in this. I imagined that I would be invited to submit an ethnographic study as a separate project in the program project grant proposal. This was not the case. At our meeting, the vice-president made his position very clear. Project CAN-DO was doomed. An eminent panel of outside reviewers, convened several months earlier, had declared it to be too diffuse an effort and had decried the lack of concrete results within the first five years of the project. I had attended that meeting and had presented my research plans there, but I had not been privy to the conclusions of the reviewers. So it came as a shock to me to hear the project declared dead. The vice-president asked my views. I offered some defense of the project and some agreement with specific criticisms. I stated that five years was only long enough to lay a groundwork for a project like Project CAN-DO. He responded by pressing me about my own training. Did I have any knowledge of medical matters? Had I taken statistics? My answers to both being affirmative, he replied that I had the kind of training that Fox Chase expected from its investigators. He pushed on, making sure that I understood exactly what he was saying. I had to understand, he said, that "ethnography is your avocation." Certainly, I had heard warnings from several quarters that ethnography was not fundable through the National Cancer Institute. The vice-president's challenge to me was clear: could I write a fundable proposal? He had, in broad outlines, a concept for a new project. It would build on another investigator's previous successes with senior citizens' groups and also draw on the plans of the Project CAN-DO principal investigator for her now-defunct renewal—which she had thought she would be writing before she left—involving primary-care physicians in the Project CAN-DO community. I left with the assignment to write a new project proposal.

I was thrilled to be respected as a doctoral-level investigator. My new status, however, was disorienting and ambiguous. The Project CAN-DO staff lived through a lengthy period of anger; the project was ending, the director leaving, and an untried investigator had been put in charge. They feared that I would not be able to write a successful proposal and keep the group together and employed. I also realized during the next few months that I, an almost unknown quantity and most certainly suspect for being an anthropologist, almost had to have been given a chance: I was writing one of only five project proposals, which would give the overall cancer-control group five chances to produce three acceptable proposals. But still, I was an investigator. Analytical distance was put on hold, as I worked seven days a week, facing a dark, secluded parking lot alone night after night, to produce a fundable proposal.

The new proposal was funded. Anger abated, people left, and new people came. I threw myself into the development of a survey instrument for the new study. I also continued to work with my ethnographic data. I was well respected, well paid, and well liked as a supervisor. But increasingly, I came to feel that I was facing a choice. Why was I doing health-education research? Why was I doing ethnography? I did not have the time or energy to develop in both fields. Who was I going to be? I had grown distant from anthropology, I felt illegitimate as a health-promotion researcher, and the siren song of the medical establishment was so sweet that I could not hear my own voice clearly. I decided that it was time for a commitment.

In the end, I chose anthropology. To redeem myself as an anthropologist, I left applied anthropology, went into an academic job, and constructed my experiences in health education as a research topic. In doing so, I hoped to leave behind all my doubts about professional legitimacy. But ironically, when I assumed my first university position, I faced questions about my legitimacy as an anthropologist. New voices challenged me: you are not a real anthropologist; you have never done pure research; you have never done traditional fieldwork overseas. Clearly, to some anthropologists, studying the European-American urban working class is not a true experience of Other and reads as a parody of legitimate anthropological practice.

Most anthropologists are familiar with this conflict. It is certainly clearly expressed in written sources describing applied practice. To document this, I reviewed a number of classic discussions of applied anthropology, and recorded direct comparisons between applied and what, for want of a better word, I will call academic anthropology; descriptors of each of these categories; and statements about what the two have in common.[3] From this review, I gleaned a list of summary oppositions that are presented in Table 4.

Two general observations are of interest. First, in the sources reviewed, it is applied anthropology that seems harder to define, more problematic, to both critics and practitioners. Second, writers have

Table 4. A Dividing Line within Anthropology

Applied Anthropology	Academic Anthropology
Profession	Discipline
Training	Education
Research	Scholarship
Method	Theory
Use of knowledge ("solely")	Production of knowledge
Human needs	Pure science
Outside world	Home
Real world	Academia
Practice	Theory
Competencies	Concerns
Skills	Perspectives
Expertise	Perception
Practical affairs	Intellectual ferment
Use of theory	Reformulation of theory
Work	Reflect ("solely")
Using anthropology	Anthropology
Active	Passive
Hard	Soft
Manual	Mental
External	Internal
Future	Past

trouble conceptualizing the dividing line between applied and academic. Nonetheless, that line is presumed to be profoundly real.

In Table 4, I have divided the list of descriptors, somewhat artificially, into three sets. The first set comprises the most common general oppositions found in my review. The second set elaborates the distinction between affairs of the mind and affairs of the world. These first two sets of terms are all drawn directly from one or more of the sources used. The third set of descriptors points to higher-order expressions of the oppositions drawn: the first four pairs of terms are my own, and the last is vocabulary used in the source material.

The division described is based on a clear distinction between practical activity and academics. This distinction has animated more than one raging debate within and about academia. In this case, applied anthropology is cast as manual labor, in a sense, and as "work" in a way that academics is not. The description of the division involved is sometimes geographical and reflects a feeling that the academy is a protected place, different from all others, in which "real" is not a value. The "outside world" is not "home" to us. The "past"—often referred to by talk about tradition—is somehow the academic's own, as well.

The academic world, then, is the world of the interiority of the mind, a world in which one can close a door and create a dream undisturbed. Never mind that such moments are in fact few and far between in academic life. The applied world, in contrast, is not the Self's exclusive own. It is a world in which the anthropologist is a commodity, and volunteers to be. Never mind that applied anthropologists are usually motivated by the same ethic of advocacy that motivates their colleagues in academia. The contrast between applied and academic may be troubled in reality. But it is clear enough in debate.

This debate, at heart, is about moral stances. Anthropologists, whether applied or academic, feel a troubled sense of moral relationship to the world. The underlying question being debated, in this distinction between applied and academic work, is, Who has moral superiority? The anthropologist who maintains and defends the world of academia as holy, as morally defensible for special and ancient reasons? Or the anthropologist who is driven by practical interests, and joins the flow of common events? Some academic anthropologists, whose position is in many ways nostalgic, react defensively to their applied colleagues, feeling that these colleagues represent an implicit threat to the viability of the academic stance. The strength of the academic/applied dichotomy speaks to the centrality of a dis-ease that besets anthropology as a whole.

In my final chapter, I will discuss the deeper implications of this. Here, I will make one practical point. Enacting this dichotomy can be destructive on an individual level to those who define themselves strongly as either academic or applied anthropologists. One danger to those who define themselves as academic anthropologists is that they may render themselves unwilling to do, or incapable of doing, applied work. This can be professionally constricting, to the individual and to the profession.[4] For those who define themselves as applied anthropologists, the dichotomy holds different dangers. Applied anthropologists run the risk of stepping into the image, formed from within academia, of what a person needs to be like to survive outside the pale. In looking for models of how to be in the applied world, we may be affected by damaging assumptions that applied anthropologists are dedicated to narrow views or are less sophisticated theoretically.[5]

This fourth conflict for applied anthropologists, then, is important for all anthropologists. The dichotomy between applied and academic anthropology sets up enormous conflict for us all, whether or not we choose to face it squarely. In my own experience, the conflict has been inescapable, in both applied and academic settings. In the applied setting, I struggled to be accepted and to cast myself *to* myself as being morally and analytically superior, by virtue of my status as an anthropologist. But in academia, there were voices in my very own field that told me that I was in fact *not* a real anthropologist at all, because I had done only applied work and only in my own society. Surely this irony harms us all. To be an applied anthropologist—in fact, to be an anthropologist at all—is to assume a very complicated self.

In my own story, familiar conflicts are replayed. Like everyone else I have described in this book, I struggled to negotiate my own place in the world in the face of professional authorities, and I lived with conflicts concerning professional control of truth, feeling, and meaning. My own struggle, like that of others, involved the question of resistance to compliance. Before me was a demand that I affiliate to medical authority. From the strength of that authority, I absorbed the desire to be respected as a competent health-education researcher and to feel ethical while advising people to hold themselves responsible for their own health. In the final analysis, I resisted and chose to resign from my position at Fox Chase. But, like everyone else, I found no escape in my resistance.

In escaping the assumption of medical authority, I faced other authorities who sought to judge me and who demanded specific forms of compliance from me. Anthropology, academic or applied, is a profession and is therefore rooted in judgment, authority, and discrimination of worthiness—although anthropologists disguise this by a thick veneer of advocacy for the less powerful and by the loudly proclaimed ethic that we are "giving the people a voice." The ugly side of authority in anthropology comes through very clearly in the way we treat each other. As is true for other professionals, being legitimate as an anthropologist demands compliance to code.

What my own story illustrates is the way in which professional authority demands compliance not only from those over whom authority is exerted but also from those who are exerting authority. The code of professional conduct in U.S. society—whether the profession be medicine, law, social work, or anthropology—centers on the assumption of authority over others. Professionals are supposed to feel comfortable, justified, and legitimate in this authority. Those over whom professional authority is exercised are described by canon as inferior or inadequate in some way—as less knowledgeable, less rational, less healthy, less well behaved, less mature, less powerful, or less insightful. The assumption of authority allows the professional to feel superior to specific others.

Professional authority is experienced in the context of many familiar relationships. Two almost inescapable such relationships are those between patient and physician and between student and teacher. These relationships need not be built on professional authority as we know it. As it is, however, we learn and teach, through these relationships and others, that it is natural to be judged. In a thousand ways in our everyday lives, we assume that we will be measured, and we fear that we will be judged insufficient, by authorities whose philosophies and standards are beyond our control. This is a fundamental experience in modern life.[6] Although we all experience both judging and being judged, and may frequently cross the line between the two, we nevertheless live with an overarching general sense of a great divide between the judges and the judged. This explains what it means to become a professional. Those who aim to do so yearn to win the authority game and to be one of the judges, or, at least, to affiliate with them. Those who earn professional status experience their new authority with considerable pride. Being one of the judges makes us feel successful. Professional authority is the opiate of the white-collar class.

If professionalism stands for success, then what stands for non-success in our society? In the story I tell here, it is working-class status. Tannerstown and the Tannerstowners Jennifer and John represent the working class. Project CAN-DO and Dr. Hughes represent the authority of the professional class over them. Neither Dr. Hughes nor the Project CAN-DO staff is motivated by overt images of social-class prejudice. But they construct their purposes and self-images with help from the concept of professional authority. In an essential sense, they thus render themselves as judges. They may do so in a way that is hidden to them. They may even seek to reject the role. But judges they are. And in our society, *the working class is a central model for the judged*. It is certainly not the only such model. Conceptions of both gender and race are independent, and both carry unique images of inequality and inferiority. Social class imagery, however, is often linked to them both. Racist images are particularly likely to be intertwined with images that refer to social class (see discussion in Reed 1992). By various means, many images of the judged—the poor, the disadvantaged, the undereducated, the disenfranchised, the ignorant—are modeled in part by images of the working class, images of what it means to fail to achieve professional status. In U.S. society, professional authority and negative (or romantic) images of the working class are essentially intermixed. Where professional is Self, the working class is Other.

Professional authority is a central underpinning of the social-class divide, a specific mechanism through which class subordination is experienced. In the present story, it is the instrument through which a working-class community is blamed for its high cancer rate; it is the instrument through which Jennifer is denied the authority to define the meaning of John's cancer. What my own story adds is that this instrument can be painful to the hand of its wielder. Professional authority victimizes both the judged and the judges. And yet, we must not count this as a tie. Tannerstowners live down the street from a chemicals plant. Most professionals do not. The distinction between working–class and professional–class status operates on physical and economic planes as well as on psychological and cultural ones.

The self-reflection on which this chapter is based has served to complicate my understanding of professional authority and to sharpen my focus on the relationship between professional authority and social class. With this as background, I will return to the question with which I began this book. That question concerns, at root, the ethics of assuming a particular professional authority over a particular working-class community.

CHANGING THE VICTIM 6

In creating a cultural hegemony, the [bourgeoisie] slowly made [its] own
culture invisible; it was seen more and more in terms of human nature or
plain common sense. Ideas about the way the world ought to be were
developed into the unquestionable facts of life. This process also affected
the missionary activities directed toward the workers and peasants. Moral
arguments increasingly gave way to scientific ones, as in the heightened
preoccupation with matters of hygiene. At the same time that bourgeois
values were becoming more and more unreflected and unconscious, the
different life-styles of others were redefined as social, medical, and
cultural deviance.

(Jonas Frykman and Orvar Löfgren, *Culture Builders* [*Den koltiverade
människan*, Sweden, 1979])

[P]ower becomes legitimate to those it wounds through the very means by
which the powerful seek to convince themselves that, faced with inferior
people, they can at least do some good.

(Richard Sennett and Jonathan Cobb, *The Hidden Injuries of Class*)

The problem that motivated this book is at root a moral dilemma of my
own. Reason tells me that there is nothing morally wrong with advising
people to change their habits to reduce their cancer risk. But when I
worked as a health educator, emotion told me that it *was* wrong. I know
from conversations with many health educators that this feeling of
moral dis-ease is common in the field. Why should this be so?

Each chapter in this book has contributed something toward an answer to this question. In this final chapter, I will review the partial answers I have given along the way and attempt to arrive at a conclusion.

COMMUNITY, CLINIC, AND ANTHROPOLOGY

In Chapter 2, I present a description of the community spirit of Tannerstown. My description is selective, stressing the community's posi-

tive spirit, its face-to-face nature, its *Gemeinschaft*. Like many classic works in social science (for instance, Gans 1962), I romanticize the European-American working class as remnants of the imagined European peasant past, thus translating a popular image into the idiom of social analysis (a mechanism discussed in Herzfeld 1987).[1] This image denigrates our imagined present in a way that serves our obsession with the ills of modernity (compare Fabian 1983). Although the image is positive, it fits with a view of Tannerstown as Other.

In Chapter 3, however, Tannerstowners represent resistance, and I interpret their rejection of health-education messages as such. I praise them for their penetrations of hegemony, their spirit of resistance, their heroism in the face of medical authority.[2] I focus on an issue of fairness: the right to allocate blame for cancer. Mainstream forces within scientific medicine claim this right; their claim is disputed by lay people who feel blamed. Given this story, where would anyone's sympathies lie? The question is loaded in favor of the community. In point of fact, most individuals who are affected by this dispute hold emotions and cognitions that are both less distinct and more complex than this bare outline would suggest. I do explore a good deal of that in this book. But the bare outline still shows through the story.

In Chapter 4, with John and Jennifer's story, I present Jennifer as a hero and give free reign to her strong and insightful voice. The story is constructed to move the reader's sympathies further along toward an appreciation of the spirit and intelligence of the community critique of medical authority. I do not present the physician, Dr. Hughes, as being immoral or insensitive. In fact, Dr. Hughes is seen as a victim, too, suffering in his own way under the yoke of medical dominance. But this does not change my presentation of Jennifer as being insightful, courageous, and motivated by a desire for justice. The closer one looks, the case study says, the more clearly one can see and feel the community's strength, and the legitimacy of the community view.

Through Chapter 4, then, this book advocates loyalty to the community position and agreement with the community critique. My own deepest loyalties lead me to this. Following Herzfeld (1987) once again, I can read this theoretical position as an academic restatement of a personal conviction. As a child at the extended family table, I learned that ordinary people are extraordinary; that we are just as smart as the highly educated; that we could get straight A's in school if we cared to; that we cannot be kept in line by the rules; and that we manipulate and defy authority if it is fun to do so. I have my own defiant ancestor, Grandpa Connors, who could quote Shakespeare, though he spent his youth riding the rails rather than sitting in school. My father, who had a college degree, could never "catch" Grandpa by finding a word he could not spell and define. The "we" that I learned to be proud of as a child was not from Tannerstown but would stand naturally on Tannerstown's side. To some significant extent, that "we" has written this book.

Thus far, I advocate a straightforward admiration of the community critique of professional authority. This does not, however, bring me all the way home. In Chapter 5, I look at authorities in my own practice and examine my own role as an anthropologist. This self-reflection, or reflexivity, is a powerful tool for anthropologists: our critical awareness of the paradoxical nature of the self-knowledge of others forces on us a parallel awareness of our own constructions of reality (Karp and Kendall 1982). When I examine my own role, I find the authority paradox that lies at the root of all anthropological practice. Anthropology is a form of practice that assumes authority by denying it. It is a practice crafted by intellectuals in rich Western nations, an identity through which people uncomfortable with privilege speak and advocate for the less privileged. But this is an assumption of authority, too. And because authority is at the root of the anthropological profession, as it is of all bourgeois professions, it is hard for anthropologists in applied settings to resist the flow of other professional authorities into our Selves. My own experience is typical: in the applied medical setting, I felt an urgent need to ward off my own assumption of medical authority.[3]

This reflexivity furthers my argument regarding the conflict between medical science and the lay public. Conflicts are often illuminated through the experience of those whose social positions and practices, in Max Gluckman's words, "cross the separation of interests"

(1958:21). As health educator and anthropologist, I played ambiguous and uncomfortable social roles in which I "crossed the separation" of many interests and identities. Following my own complex role leads me, in Chapter 5, to understand clearly that the satisfactions of our professional authorities must be undone before social class domination will look like what it is.

But reflexivity furthers my purpose in a second way. Through reflexivity, I seek to cure my enduring dis-ease. The story of Tannerstown, the story of John and Jennifer, and the story of my life as a health educator all serve to illuminate a web of professional authority, working-class resistance, and social-class conflict. But my telling of my own story also serves as my attempt to disentangle myself from this web. In this book, I display my struggle to shed the professional authorities I learned, both in graduate school and at Fox Chase, and my attempt to construct an anthropological authority that feels moral. My construction of the other professionals with whom I worked serves this attempt. Faced with the lure to affiliate with medical authority, I negotiate a sense of independent Self through a critique of the professional practice of Others. I construct a view of myself, for myself, as the only real advocate for the community. My analysis is designed to reproduce for me the assertions I most need to hear: that I am in fact truly an anthropologist and that anthropology is in fact truly a moral enterprise. My self-reflection continues this process to the core. In this sense, this book is a confession, a cleansing, a process of atonement.

In more or less direct ways, each chapter of this book points toward my central question as being a question of ethics. I have structured the story of the book to create admiration for the intelligence of the community, empathy for the sufferings of John and Jennifer, and insight concerning professional authority and class discrimination. My self-reflection also stands as an attempt to escape from an assumption of authority that I ultimately feel to be unacceptable. This all casts doubts on the general question of the morality of professional authority. As my self-reflection indicates, my ethnography is structured this way because my discourse is motivated at the root by my own sense of moral discomfort.

THE TAKE-HOME MESSAGE

In the final analysis, how do I answer my central question? Why did it feel illegitimate to me to advise people to change their lifestyles in order to reduce their risk of cancer? Through writing this book, my own emotional reactions have become clearer to me, and my answer has become grounded in my understanding of professional authority.

It did *not* feel morally wrong to me to advise people to stop smoking. It *did* feel morally wrong to do so from a judgmental perspective. And it is hard to be a health educator or a physician without participating in the judging that is an essential part of modern forms of professional authority. I now feel free to see it as defensible, and desirable, to help people stop smoking. I do not see it as defensible to do so from within frameworks that assume a transmittal of truth and authority from professionals to lay people.

Health educators teach more than their literal message. They also teach the rightness of the prevailing social relations between the medical profession and the lay public. The message that this transmits, the one that is hard for all concerned to live with, is, "accept authority and accept blame." This message has a social reality that is as deep as that of the literal message to quit smoking, go for a checkup, or the like. It is based on an assumption of professional worldviews as superior and on master images of inferiority—such as the image of the working class, which is the image I have explored here.[4] Like the residents of Tannerstown, I saw the literal message as being transformed by the social relations through which it was transmitted. No amount of "cultural sensitivity" in health-education practice will speak to this root problem. The world of the message makers needs fundamental change.

As I have noted, this point is not new to the literature in health promotion. In many schools, students of health education or health promotion are taught that it is ideal to let communities and patients set their own priorities for educational and other service programs. Influential scholars in health promotion and health education have taken a stand against victim blaming and in favor of a more environmental model of disease causation and health behavior. Scholars such as Meredith Minkler and Nina Wallerstein have written on these issues with great insight and passion; similar concerns are established among medical practitioners.

To the dismay of many in both health promotion and clinical medicine, however, awareness has not translated well into practice. If this book is useful to practitioners in either profession—or to professional anthropologists—it will be because it stands as documentation of how difficult it is to confront the professional authorities within. I have written on health education, medicine, and anthropology, the professions I know best: I suspect that the same basic problems face all professions. This book stands as a case study of the subtle bonds of professional authority on judges and judged alike. Clearly, profound personal and cultural transformations are necessary before academic ideals about community and patient self-determination can be realized in professional practice.

Project CAN-DO is a case in point. It is the greatest of ironies that Project CAN-DO should have participated in and been informed by a judgmental professional paradigm. Project leadership and field staff opposed such thinking and struggled to overcome it. But the paradigm was asserted because it was dominant among the higher authorities to which the project staff was accountable and because it is so difficult to imagine alternative forms of professional practice. We moved from "myth" to "misconception" but could move no further. We did not escape the framework in which the ideas of Others are seen as oppositional, adversarial, and in some sense inferior to our own.

My purpose is not to turn the tables and blame the judges. I have tried to portray the professionals in this book—the Project CAN-DO staff, Dr. Hughes, and myself—as both authorities and victims. Many people in the professions I describe feel the judgmental basis of their practice, suffer in the role of judge, and position themselves as advocates to avoid feeling their assumptions of authority. All the professionals in this book—health educator, physician, and anthropologist— claim to be not authorities but advocates.[5] But we all assume authority nonetheless. Anthropologists are perhaps the most trenchant example of this—claiming at the same time to renounce authority and to possess a legitimate truth. This dilemma is absolutely fundamental to anthropology, whether phenomenology or reflexivity is counted as the path to truth. Those who deny this are in effect making unseen the authorities entailed in the ethnographic stance (see Karp and Kendall 1982:269).

But what is to be done? How is professional practice to be reformed? William Ryan offers a succinct statement of the program recommended by a judgmental professional stance: "The formula for action becomes extraordinarily simple: change the victim" (1976 :8). This is a program that must be profoundly rejected. Anthropologists, like all professionals, must work past the tacit tendency to define Others as problematic. Such conceptual frameworks support policy and programmatic practice that reproduces power differences between social classes and accentuates the pain and conflict that these differences engender. If nothing else, such practice is likely to be ineffective. The people of Tannerstown do not want or need our diagnosis. They are insisting as loudly as they can that we attend to the real problem, which is the terms of our conflict with them. In the final analysis, they are right. We need to stop thinking about transforming Other lives. The best take-home advice—for health educators, physicians, and anthropologists alike—is that when we think about changing the victim, we should think about changing ourselves.

NOTES

Preface

1. Brown and Margo (1978) present a strong, early critique of health education, asking if the "reformers" can be "reformed." Leventhal, Meyer, and Gutman (1980) present a powerful argument against use of the concept of the culture of poverty. Minkler and Pasick (1986), writing on the tendency to blame the elderly for their health problems, deconstruct the notion of responsibility for health, suggesting that we focus instead on "response-ability." In a later statement Minkler (1989) argues against the focus on change in personal behavior and for a focus on empowerment and environmental factors. This article is an excellent review of the basic issues involved, by an important figure in the field. Wallerstein and Bernstein (1988), drawing on the work of Paulo Freire (1971), write in favor of the "empowerment education" approach for health education. Blaming the victim is also critiqued in McLeroy et al. (1988) and, with specific regard to cancer control, by Eriksen (1989). In a series of important and stimulating articles, Pill and Stott (1982, 1985, 1987) offer a critique of the concept of working-class fatalism. Also related is the argument that community organizing should replace education in community health work. Bowser et al. (1990) make a strong statement of this view, offering suggestions for concrete strategies. Farrant (1991) offers a thought-provoking historical review of the reaction against victim blaming; Brown (1991) gives a particularly clear

conceptual statement. Also relevant to these issues is the literature on the training of lay volunteers in health promotion campaigns (see, for instance, Roberson 1987). This review is by no means exhaustive, but it serves to indicate the importance of critical perspectives within the field of health education itself. Similar perspectives are also established in clinical medicine. Many physicians have written about medical dominance and their own desires to transform power relations in the practice of medicine. Well-known examples include H. Aoun (1992); Eric J. Cassell (1976); David Hilfiker (1985); and Kerr L. White (1988).

CHAPTER 1. DEFINING THE TOPIC

1. This creation of analytical distance is basic for academics. It forms a private space and a relationship with the world within which academics feel secure. The sense of commitment that many academics feel to analytical frameworks—often referred to as "theoretical positions"—springs from a strong need to secure this safe space.

2. Actually, most descriptions of working-class life draw from both sides of this somewhat unfortunate debate. Descriptions of the working class are more appropriately seen as lying on a continuum, with individual authors rendering either structural constraints or working-class resistance more dramatically. For instance, Belle (1982) focuses on the debilitating emotional effect of poverty in the lives of low-income mothers; whereas Martin (1987) focuses on the spirit of women who resist the dominance of scientific medicine. But each account shows us both spirit and economics. Other well-balanced accounts are presented by Irwin and Jordan (1987) and Rapp (1988).

3. It is clearly and abundantly documented by the literature that working-class people are less likely to use preventive health services and less likely to conform to recommendations regarding lifestyle changes for health promotion. Two main types of explanations for this are advanced. Some point to practical barriers, such as access or financial issues. In practice, the removal of such barriers is hardly ever sufficient to change health behaviors. Others point to health beliefs as having a strong influence. In the field of health promotion, the Health Belief Model is a key and seminal framework (see Becker 1974; Hochbaum 1958; Janz and Becker 1984; Rosenstock 1966, 1974). Many good discussions of social-class differences in health status and health behavior assign importance to both practical and attitudinal factors (for example, Calnan and Johnson 1985; Rundall and Wheeler 1979; and Wing 1988).

Still, by and large, most discussions of health beliefs and behaviors stand on the assumption that some people possess bad behaviors and attitudes and that we need to change those people for the better.

4. The basic literature on compliance is reviewed in Becker and Maimon 1975 and Leventhal and Cameron 1987. This literature is vast and covers the problem of the noncompliance of patients with recommendations from physicians, and general noncompliance with recommendations for prevention. Much of this literature strives to be nonjudgmental. Some have suggested replacing the word *compliance* with terms such as *adherence,* which implies dialogue and consensus. Leventhal, Meyer, and Gutmann (1980) present such an argument, directly criticizing compliance models that assume "attitude and knowledge malfunctions" (1980:11–12) in noncompliers. This is progressive but not paradigmatic. The bottom-line goal is still that "they" conform to what "we" advise. I would compare this to Taussig's discussion of the "illusion of reciprocity" created by the "packaging of 'care,' 'trust,' and 'feelings' " (1980:23) in clinical practice. As Trostle points out in a discussion of patient manipulation and terminology: "The word 'compliant' has unfortunate connotations, but the underlying concept also needs reworking" (1988:1306). The case study presented by Taussig (1980) and the discussion by Singer (1987) are also relevant to a critique of the simple behaviorist interpretation of compliance.

CHAPTER 2. THE STUDY COMMUNITY

1. The history summarized here is covered in Binzen 1970; Duffy 1982; Mallowe 1986; and Randall and Soloman 1977.

2. Material presented later in this chapter leads me to speculate on the extent to which being "poor and white," through some racist enigma, may seem particularly offensive to the predominantly European-American professional world in the United States.

3. Using data on cancer mortality for the United States, Philadelphia, and the Tannerstown neighborhood, I was able to corroborate most of this picture; however, data for Tannerstown were too limited to allow for a reliable analysis. Data on cancer mortality by age group for the United States can be found in the Department of Health and Human Services publication, issued yearly, entitled *Health United States.* I used the 1991 edition (U.S. Centers for Disease Control 1991). Some of the data I used for Philadelphia and Tannerstown were supplied by the State Health Data Center, Pennsylvania Department of Health, Harrisburg,

Pennsylvania. The department specifically disclaims responsibility for any analysis, interpretations, or conclusions.

4. Various approaches to the study of the possible link between air pollution and cancer are reported in Doll 1989; Freeman and Cattell 1988; Lewtas and Gallagher 1990; and Richters 1988. Doll's essay is a particularly clear and intelligent statement, from an eminent authority, of the very conservative tone of much of this research. Discussions of cancer and air pollution are also found in Epstein 1978 and Goldsmith 1980.

5. The same type of humor is found in Fussell 1983, who speaks derisively of every social class and then puts himself and his supposedly sophisticated readers in "category 'X.' " He explains that "in discovering that you can become an X person you find the only escape from class" (1983:212–13). The illustrations in Fussell's book (see, for instance, 1983:49, 63) show his contempt for working-class people in particular.

6. Many of the "by Dan" columns in my collection were clipped for me during 1986–88, when I worked for Project CAN-DO. Unfortunately, many of these clippings are not dated, and I have been unable to date them using editions of the *Guide* available at the Free Library of Philadelphia. Where I have dates for "by Dan" columns, I cite them in these notes. Where no date is available, there is no citation.

7. May 19, 1988.

8. March 1, 1979.

9. July 16, 1987.

10. May 7, 1987.

11. August 18, 1988.

12. April 5, 1979.

13. June 10, 1988.

CHAPTER 3. PROJECT CAN-DO

1. The concept and title for this fictive panel was the creation of Martha Kasper Keintz. The stories offered here as illustration are not her responsibility.

2. Permission to quote was given by Arthur Betcher, who, with his wife, Mary, wrote this memorial for their beloved daughter, Linda M. Goodwin, who died of cancer at the age of forty. Arthur Betcher agreed to quotation of this material in the hope that it would help physicians and researchers understand the sorrow felt by families that lose a loved one to cancer.

3. A vast qualitative literature documents this (see Balshem 1988; Belle 1982; Binzen 1970; Garson 1975; Rubin 1976; Sacks and Remy 1984; Shostak 1980; Tepperman 1976; Willis 1977; and reviews in Balshem 1985 and Burowoy 1979). It is also documented in health promotion research, using quantitative variables such as self-efficacy and locus of health control. Peterson and Stunkard (1989) present an important statement on the centrality of beliefs about control to the process of health-care decision making. They assert the importance of understanding social context in this regard.

4. An analysis of community discourse about heart disease is beyond the scope of this discussion. In general, however, in the United States, both medical and lay beliefs about heart disease tend to be tied to a stress model. This model describes the individual heart disease process as a material synecdoche for the everyday harshness of modern life, particularly work life (see, for instance, Eyer 1975; French and Caplan 1970; Haynes et al. 1980; Karasek et al. 1981; Rosenman et al. 1975; Scotch 1963). This entails a focus on the individual disease process that may depoliticize perceptions of the social causation of heart disease, but the process is subtle, and there is assonance between lay and scientific rhetoric (cf. Young 1980). In any case, in Tannerstown, cancer is much better suited to carry the sentiments of resistance I have described here. This is not to say that heart disease might not do so in different circumstances (see British Broadcasting Corporation 1991).

5. For example, see Adonis 1978; Antonovsky 1972; Dent and Goulston 1982; EVAXX 1981; Gordon 1990; Long and Long 1982; Michielutte and Diseker 1982; National Cancer Institute 1986; Ragucci 1981; Saillant 1990; Salzberger 1976; Sontag 1977. I would reiterate the point that Tannerstowners are not unique in expressing these images of cancer. Their expression of these images, however, tied as it is to dramatic local circumstances that bring to the fore feelings about cancer, is elaborate and profound. In particular, Tannerstowners openly relate their talk about cancer to a wider discourse on control and authority. I strongly suspect that this relation, although often less obviously expressed, informs images of cancer beyond the boundaries of Tannerstown, as well.

6. See Balshem et al. 1988; Celentano and Holtzman 1983; Greenwald 1980; Knopf 1976; Minkler 1981; National Cancer Institute 1986; Rimer et al. 1983. This literature fits into the enormous body of work, cited earlier, documenting the general tendency of those of lower socioeconomic status to forgo preventive medical care.

7. Residents sometimes state that they have already changed their health habits (for instance, reduced dietary fat or quit smoking) in order to

prevent heart disease, but they resist advice to make the same or similar changes in order to prevent cancer (see discussion of this mechanism in Ben-Sira 1977). Of course, the extent to which residents have actually changed their health habits, for whatever reason, cannot be assessed in my study.

CHAPTER 4. A CANCER DEATH

1. I present both Jennifer's story and the medical record more or less chronologically. Quotations from both documents are interspersed, but the line of Jennifer's story is preserved—that is, the quotations from the first interview with Jennifer are presented in the order in which they were originally said.

2. The first procedure was an exploratory laparotomy; a constricting lesion of the terminal ileum and ascending colon was resected. The second procedure was a decompressive laminectomy of the eighth and ninth thoracic vertebrae, with gross residual disease noted. The surgical pathology report from the laminectomy specified a diagnosis of a poorly differentiated carcinoma.

3. The autopsy report lists bilateral bronchopneumonia as the direct cause of death, with the antecedent cause listed as "carcinomatosis due to carcinoma of tail of pancreas." Metastasis was extensive. Jennifer's report that "[t]hey'd never seen [that kind of cancer] before" should not be taken to mean that Hospital F had never treated a case of pancreatic cancer; what this remark does refer to is unclear. Jennifer also raises the question of whether John's physicians prescribed the right chemotherapy for him. His chemotherapy program consisted of Cytoxan, Adriamycin, and 5-fluorouracil, a broad and aggressive treatment for an unknown primary tumor, thought most likely to be oat cell carcinoma of the lung. It is highly unlikely that a chemotherapy program designed for treatment of pancreatic cancer would have produced any more than the transient benefit that was produced by the program that was followed. It should be noted that the course of John's disease was not unusual. Pancreatic cancer is typically discovered late and has a very poor prognosis. In the early stages of the disease, there are often no symptoms. The first symptoms to appear—John's back pain and indigestion being common—are very frequently diagnosed as something else, such as happened in John's case. The earliest symptoms may be caused by metastatic tumors. In cancers of the tail of the pancreas,

pain often does not appear until late in the course of the disease—usually too late, in fact, for effective treatment.

CHAPTER 5. MEANING FOR THE ANTHROPOLOGIST

1. On the topic of reflexivity in anthropology, the following references are important: Fabian 1983; Herzfeld 1987; Karp and Kendall 1982; Said 1978. In the widely read volume edited by Clifford and Marcus (1986), the articles by Rosaldo and Clifford are especially valuable.
2. As I emphasized earlier, my critique of health education falls within a well-established and central debate in that field, in which the field's traditional focus on lifestyle and individual responsibility for health are soundly criticized.
3. The following works were included in my review: Chambers 1985: chaps. 1, 6, and 7; Chambers 1987; Eddy and Partridge 1987: preface and introduction; Goldschmidt 1979: introduction; van Willigen 1986; and Wulff and Fiske 1987. I also reviewed all 1990 and 1991 issues of the newsletter of the Society for Applied Anthropology; these were not a rich source for my search. This list of sources is by no means exhaustive, but it represents a sampling of some basic statements about applied anthropology.
4. I will point to an example from my own experience. In one instance, I worked on a short-term project in applied anthropology with a very able and experienced colleague who openly defined himself as an academic anthropologist. His agonized discourse about applied work covered many issues. But what he talked about most was time. Time constraints meant work, in an alienated sense, and he could not bear to put his insight and creativity into that box. He was also haunted by the fact that his work would have a direct and immediate effect on policy. This threatened his sense that his primary relationship with his informants was one of genuine caring. He needed to prove to his readership, including himself, that he was more than an anthropologist to the people with whom he worked. These concerns rendered him incapable of finishing the project—a loss to both the project and, in my view, to him.
5. Images of work in applied sociocultural anthropology are paralleled in considerable detail by images of contract work in archaeology. This was pointed out to me by Stephen C. Hamilton and other students at a Portland State University Anthropology Students Association meeting in March 1992.

6. This insight is being developed by Rosemary Wray Williams in her continuing work on the discourse of assessment in education.

CHAPTER 6. CHANGING THE VICTIM

1. Health educators, too, sometimes describe a community like Tannerstown as being of the past. In one instance, a health educator hired to work in a neighborhood similar to Tannerstown was told that when one works in such a neighborhood, one has to turn the clock back twenty years. Another health educator, also working in a similar neighborhood, spoke of the "June Cleaver Model for Health Education." Yet another health educator, musing on the residents of a similar European-American working-class neighborhood, expressed the following: "I think they brought with them a lot of the feelings that they had in Europe when they migrated, and one of those things was a general disrespect for organized medicine, and, um—they relied on themselves for health care, and um—so I think that's just a tradition that's been handed down." As these images make clear, many health educators see places such as Tannerstown as being holdovers—from the 1950s or from the peasants of Europe—who belong to a past in which people still had faith in patriarchal institutions.
2. I look for them to be more heroic than I myself feel.
3. I believe this experience to be typical, partly on the basis of reactions to a paper I presented at an American Anthropological Association meeting (Balshem 1991b).
4. As noted above, there are other master images of inferiority that have autonomous, although usually intertwined, existences. Images based on racial inferiority and on gender are the obvious examples.
5. In fact, every major character in this book, including the patient's wife, claims to be an advocate for community, patient, or both. I am indebted to Ivan Karp for this insight.

REFERENCES

Adonis, Catherine
1978   "French Cultural Attitudes towards Cancer." *Cancer Nursing* 1:111–
        13.
Amsel, Zili, Andrew M. Balshem, Doris Gillespie, Prakash Grover, and
    Paul F. Engstrom
1986   "Cancer Related Attitudes and Practices in a Community Experienc-
        ing High Cancer Mortality." In *Advances in Cancer Control: Health
        Care Financing and Research*. Lee E. Mortenson, Paul F. Engstrom,
        and Paul N. Anderson, eds., pp. 247–61. New York: Alan R. Liss.
Antonovsky, Aaron
1972   "The Image of Four Diseases Held by the Urban Jewish Population
        of Israel." *Journal of Chronic Diseases* 25:375–84.
Aoun, H.
1992   "From the Eye of the Storm, with the Eyes of a Physician." *Annals
        of Internal Medicine* 116 (4):335–38.
Balshem, Martha
1985   "Job Stress and Health among Women Clerical Workers." Ph.D.
        dissertation, Department of Anthropology, Indiana University.
1988   "The Clerical Worker's Boss: An Agent of Job Stress." *Human Orga-
        nization* 47:361–67.
1991a   "Cancer, Control, and Causality: Talking about Cancer in a
        Working-Class Community." *American Ethnologist* 18:152–72.
1991b   "A Critical Analysis of an Applied Medical Setting." Paper pre-

sented at the 90th Annual Meeting of the American Anthropological Association, November 20, Chicago.

Balshem, Martha, Zili Amsel, Stephen Workman, and Andrew Balshem

1986 "Attitudes towards Cancer in a High Cancer Mortality Community." Paper presented at the 85th Annual Meeting of the American Anthropological Association, December 4, Philadelphia.

Balshem, Martha, Zili Amsel, Stephen Workman, Andrew Balshem, and Paul F. Engstrom

1988 "Development of a Nutrition Education Program for a Blue Collar Community." In *Advances in Cancer Control: Cancer Control Research and the Emergence of the Oncology Product Line.* Paul F. Engstrom, Paul N. Anderson, and Lee E. Mortenson, eds., pp. 65–76. New York: Alan R. Liss.

Becker, Marshall H., ed.

1974 *The Health Belief Model and Personal Health Behavior.* Special issue. *Health Education Monographs* 2 (4).

Becker, Marshall H., and Lois A. Maiman

1975 "Sociobehavioral Determinants of Compliance with Health and Medical Care Recommendations." *Medical Care* 13 (1):10–24.

Belle, Deborah, ed.

1982 *Lives in Stress: Women and Depression.* Beverly Hills: Sage Publications.

Ben-Sira, Zeev

1977 "Involvement with a Disease and Health-promoting Behavior." *Social Science and Medicine* 11:165–73.

Binzen, Peter

1970 *Whitetown, U.S.A.* New York: Vintage Books, Random House.

Bowser, Benjamin P., Mindy Thompson Fullilove, and Robert E. Fullilove

1990 "African-American Youth and AIDS High-risk Behavior: The Social Context and Barriers to Prevention." *Youth and Society* 22 (1):54–66.

British Broadcasting Corporation

1991 *Half-hearted about Semi-skimmed.* Tessa Livingstone, producer. Transcription of BBC Horizon science series broadcast transmitted June 24. London: British Broadcasting Corporation.

Brown, E. Richard

1991 "Community Action for Health Promotion: A Strategy to Empower Individuals and Communities." *International Journal of Health Services* 21 (3):441–56.

Brown, E. Richard, and Glen Elgin Margo

1978 "Health Education: Can the Reformers Be Reformed?" *International Journal of Health Services* 8 (1):3–26.

Burawoy, Michael

1979   "The Anthropology of Industrial Work." *Annual Review of Anthropology* 8:231–66.

Calnan, Michael, and Barbara Johnson

1985   "Health, Health Risks, and Inequalities: An Exploratory Study of Women's Perceptions." *Sociology of Health and Illness* 7 (1):55–75.

Cassell, Eric J.

1976   *The Healer's Art*. Cambridge, Mass.: MIT Press.

Celentano, David D., and Deborah Holtzman

1983   "Breast Self-examination Competency: An Analysis of Self-reported Practice and Associated Characteristics." *American Journal of Public Health* 73:1321–23.

Chambers, Erve

1985   *Applied Anthropology: A Practical Guide*. Prospect Heights, Ill.: Waveland Press.

1987   "Applied Anthropology in the Post-Vietnam Era: Anticipations and Ironies." *Annual Review of Anthropology* 16:309–37.

Cicourel, Aaron V.

1983   "Language and the Structure of Belief in Medical Communication." In *The Social Organization of Doctor-Patient Communication*. Sue Fisher and Alexandra Dundas Todd, eds., pp. 221–39. Washington, D.C.: Center for Applied Linguistics.

Clifford, James

1986   "On Ethnographic Allegory." In *Writing Culture: The Poetics and Politics of Ethnography*. James Clifford and George E. Marcus, eds., pp. 98–121. Berkeley: University of California Press.

Clifford, James, and George E. Marcus, eds.

1986   *Writing Culture: The Poetics and Politics of Ethnography*. Berkeley: University of California Press.

Dayal, Hari, Chung Yin Chiu, Robert Sharrar, John Mangan, Ira Rosenwaike, Stuart Shapiro, A. J. Henley, Robert Goldberg-Alberts, and Judith Kinman

1984   "Ecologic Correlates of Cancer Mortality Patterns in an Industrialized Urban Population." *Journal of the National Cancer Institute* 73 (3):565–74.

Dent, Owen, and Kerry Goulston

1982   "Community Attitudes to Cancer." *Journal of Biosocial Science* 14:359–72.

DiGiacomo, Susan M.

1992   "Metaphor as Illness: Postmodern Dilemmas in the Representation of Body, Mind, and Disorder." *Medical Anthropology* 14:109–37.

Doll, R.

1989   "Mineral Fibres in the Non-occupational Environment: Concluding Remarks." In *Non-occupational Exposure to Mineral Fibres*. J. Bignon, J. Peto, and R. Saracci, eds., pp. 511–18. Lyons, France: International Agency for Research on Cancer.

Doll, Richard, and Richard Peto

1981   *The Causes of Cancer: Quantitative Estimates of Avoidable Risks of Cancer in the United States Today*. Oxford: Oxford University Press.

Duffy, Glen

1982   "Bridesburg Stinks!" *Philadelphia Magazine* 73 (12):132–34, 170–82.

Eddy, Elizabeth M., and William L. Partridge, eds.

1987   *Applied Anthropology in America*. 2d edition. New York: Columbia University Press.

Epstein, Samuel S.

1978   *The Politics of Cancer*. San Francisco: Sierra Club Books.

Eriksen, Michael P.

1989   "Emerging Issues in Cancer Control." *Health Education Research* 4 (4):501–505.

EVAXX, Inc.

1981   *A Study of Black Americans' Attitudes toward Cancer and Cancer Tests: Highlights*. New York: American Cancer Society.

Eyer, Joseph

1975   "Hypertension as a Disease of Modern Society." *International Journal of Health Services* 5 (4):539–58.

Fabian, Johannes

1983   *Time and the Other: How Anthropology Makes Its Object*. New York: Columbia University Press.

Fackelmann, Kathy A.

1990   "Air Pollution Boosts Cancer Spread." *Science News* 137 (14):221.

Farquhar, John W., Nathan Maccoby, Peter D. Wood, Janet K. Alexander, Henry Breitrose, Byron W. Brown, Jr., William L. Haskell, Alfred L. McAlister, Anthony J. Meyer, Joyce D. Nash, and Michael P. Stern

1977   "Community Education for Cardiovascular Health." *Lancet* 8023:1192–95.

Farrant, Wendy

1991   "Addressing the Contradictions: Health Promotion and Community Health Action in the United Kingdom." *International Journal of Health Services* 21 (3):423–39.

Fortes, Meyer

1987   "Coping with Destiny." In *Religion, Morality, and the Person: Essays on Tallensi Religion.* Jack Goody, ed., pp. 145–74. New York: Cambridge University Press.

Freeman, Diana J., and Frank C. R. Cattell
1988   "The Risk of Lung Cancer from Polycyclic Aromatic Hydrocarbons in Sydney Air." *Medical Journal of Australia* 149:612–15.

Freire, Paulo
1971   *Pedagogy of the Oppressed.* Myra Bergman Ramos, transl. New York: Herder and Herder. (Original: *Pedagogia del oprimido,* Portugal, 1968.)

French, John R. P., Jr., and Robert D. Caplan
1970   "Psychosocial Factors in Coronary Heart Disease." *Industrial Medicine* 39 (9):31–45.

Fussell, Paul
1983   *Class.* New York: Ballantine Books.

Gale, Debby, Mindy Kitei, and Ronnie Polaneczky, eds.
1982   "Philadelphia Style Goes to the Shore." *Philadelphia Magazine* 73 (8):104–109.

Gans, Herbert J.
1962   *The Urban Villagers: Group and Class in the Life of Italian-Americans.* New York: Free Press.

Garson, Barbara
1975   *All the Livelong Day: The Meaning and Demeaning of Routine Work.* Garden City, N.Y.: Doubleday.

Gluckman, Max
1958   *Analysis of a Social Situation in Modern Zululand.* The Rhodes-Livingstone Papers, no. 28. Manchester, England: Manchester University Press.

Goldschmidt, Walter, ed.
1979   *The Uses of Anthropology.* Washington, D.C.: American Anthropological Association.

Goldsmith, John R.
1980   "The 'Urban Factor' in Cancer: Smoking, Industrial Exposures, and Air Pollution as Possible Explanations." *Journal of Environmental Pathology and Toxicology* 3:205–17.

Gordon, Deborah R.
1990   "Embodying Illness, Embodying Cancer." *Culture, Medicine, and Psychiatry* 14 (2):275–97.

Greene, Michele G., Ronald Adelman, Rita Charon, and Susie Hoffman
1986   "Ageism in the Medical Encounter: An Exploratory Study of the Doctor-Elderly Patient Relationship." *Language and Communication* 6 (1/2):113–24.

Greenwald, Howard P.
1980   *Social Problems in Cancer Control.* Cambridge, Mass.: Ballinger.
Greenwald, Peter, and Edward J. Sondik, eds.
1986   "Cancer Control Objectives for the Nation: 1985–2000." NCI
        Monographs, no. 2. Division of Cancer Prevention and Control,
        National Cancer Institute, Washington, D.C.
Haynes, Suzanne G., Manning Feinleib, and William B. Kannel
1980   "The Relationship of Psychosocial Factors to Coronary Heart Dis-
        ease in the Framingham Study: III. Eight Year Incidence of Coro-
        nary Heart Disease." *American Journal of Epidemiology* 111 (1):37–58.
Herzfeld, Michael
1987   *Anthropology through the Looking-glass: Critical Ethnography in the Mar-
        gins of Europe.* New York: Cambridge University Press.
Hilfiker, David
1985   *Healing the Wounds: A Physician Looks at His Work.* New York: Pan-
        theon Books.
Hochbaum, Godfrey M.
1958   *Public Participation in Medical Screening Programs: A Socio-psychological
        Study.* Public Health Service Publication, no. 572. Washington,
        D.C.: U.S. Government Printing Office.
Illich, Ivan
1977   *Medical Nemesis: The Expropriation of Health.* Toronto: Bantam
        Books.
Irwin, Susan, and Brigitte Jordan
1987   "Knowledge, Practice, and Power: Court-ordered Cesarean Sec-
        tions." *Medical Anthropology Quarterly* 1:319–34.
Janz, Nancy K., and Marshall H. Becker
1984   "The Health Belief Model: A Decade Later." *Health Education Quar-
        terly* 11 (1):1–47.
Janzen, John M.
1978   *The Quest for Therapy: Medical Pluralism in Lower Zaire.* Berkeley:
        University of California Press.
Johannsen, Agneta M.
1992   "Applied Anthropology and Post-Modernist Ethnography." *Human
        Organization* 51:71–81.
Jordan, Bridgette
1977   "The Self-diagnosis of Early Pregnancy: An Investigation of Lay
        Competence." *Medical Anthropology* 1:1–38.
Karasek, Robert A., Dean Baker, Frank Marxer, Anders Ahlbom, and
    Tores Theorell
1981   "Job Decision Latitude, Job Demands, and Cardiovascular Disease:

A Prospective Study of Swedish Men." *American Journal of Public Health* 71:694–705.

Karp, Ivan, and Martha B. Kendall

1982   "Reflexivity in Field Work." In *Explaining Human Behavior: Consciousness, Human Action and Social Structure.* Paul F. Secord, ed., pp. 249–73. Beverly Hills: Sage Publications.

Kitei, Mindy, and the *Philadelphia Magazine* staff

1984   "Tying the Knot Philly Style." *Philadelphia Magazine* 75 (6):132–37.

Kleinman, Arthur

1980   *Patients and Healers in the Context of Culture: An Exploration of the Borderline between Anthropology, Medicine, and Psychiatry.* Berkeley: University of California Press.

1981   "The Meaning Context of Illness and Care: Reflections on a Central Theme in the Anthropology of Medicine." In *Sciences and Cultures: Anthropological and Historical Studies of the Sciences.* Everett Mendelsohn and Yehuda Elkana, eds., pp. 161–76. Dordrecht: D. Reidel.

Kleinman, Arthur, Leon Eisenberg, and Byron Good

1978   "Culture, Illness, and Care: Clinical Lessons from Anthropologic and Cross-cultural Research." *Annals of Internal Medicine* 88 (2):251–58.

Knopf, A.

1976   "Women's Beliefs about the Causes of Cancer." In *Public Education about Cancer.* J. Wakefield, ed., pp. 52–61. Geneva: UICC (International Union against Cancer).

Kornfield, Ruth

1986   "'My Belly Button Hurts': Translating Zairian Terminology into the Biomedical Framework." Paper presented at the 85th Annual Meeting of the American Anthropological Association, December 4, Philadelphia.

Leventhal, Howard, and Linda Cameron

1987   "Behavioral Theories and the Problem of Compliance." *Patient Education and Counseling* 10 (2):117–38.

Leventhal, Howard, Daniel Meyer, and Mary Gutmann

1980   "The Role of Theory in the Study of Compliance to High Blood Pressure Regimens." In *Patient Compliance to Prescribed Antihypertensive Medication Regimens: A Report to the National Heart, Lung and Blood Institute.* R. Brian Haynes, Margaret E. Mattson, and Tilmer O. Engebretson, Jr., eds., pp. 1–58. NIH Publication, no. 81–2102. Washington, D.C.: U.S. Department of Health and Human Services.

Lewtas, J., and J. Gallagher

1990   "Complex Mixtures of Urban Air Pollutants: Identification and Comparative Assessment of Mutagenic and Tumorigenic Chemicals and Emission Sources." In *Complex Mixtures and Cancer Risk.* H. Vainio, M. Sorsa, and A. J. McMichael, eds., pp. 252–60. Lyons, France: International Agency for Research on Cancer.

Lipset, Seymour Martin, and William Schneider

1983   *The Confidence Gap: Business, Labor, and Government in the Public Mind.* New York: Free Press.

Long, Susan O., and Bruce D. Long

1982   "Curable Cancers and Fatal Ulcers: Attitudes toward Cancer in Japan." *Social Science and Medicine* 16:2101–2108.

McLeroy, Kenneth R., Daniel Bibeau, Allan Steckler, and Karen Glanz

1988   "An Ecological Perspective on Health Promotion Programs." *Health Education Quarterly* 15 (4):351–77.

Mallowe, Mike

1979   "Whitetown Blues." *Philadelphia Magazine* 70 (2):88–92, 238–45.

1986   "Notes from the New White Ghetto." *Philadelphia Magazine* 77 (12):165–69, 241–50.

Martin, Emily

1987   *The Woman in the Body: A Cultural Analysis of Reproduction.* Boston: Beacon Press.

1988   "The Cultural Construction of Gendered Bodies: Biology and Metaphors of Production and Destruction." Paper presented at the Vega Day Symposium in Honor of Fredrik Barth, Swedish Society for Anthropology and Geography, April 25, Stockholm, Sweden.

1989   "Discussion. Author Meets Critics: Emily Martin and the Cultural Construction of Scientific Knowledge." Paper presented at the 88th Annual Meeting of the American Anthropological Association, November 17, Washington, D.C.

Michielutte, Robert, and Robert A. Diseker

1982   "Racial Differences in Knowledge of Cancer: A Pilot Study." *Social Science and Medicine* 16:245–52.

Minkler, Meredith

1981   "Applications of Social Support Theory to Health Education: Implications for Work with the Elderly." *Health Education Quarterly* 8 (2):147–65.

1989   "Health Education, Health Promotion and the Open Society: An Historical Perspective." *Health Education Quarterly* 16 (1):17–30.

Minkler, Meredith, and Rena J. Pasick

1986   "Health Promotion and the Elderly: A Critical Perspective on the

Past and Future." In *Wellness and Health Promotion for the Elderly*. Ken Dychtwald, ed., pp. 39–54. Rockville, Md.: Aspen Systems Corporation.

National Cancer Institute

1986   *Cancer Prevention Awareness Survey: Wave II*. Technical Report. Office of Cancer Communication. Bethesda, Md.: National Institutes of Health.

Newman, Katherine S.

1989   *Falling from Grace: The Experience of Downward Mobility in the American Middle Class*. New York: Vintage Books, Random House.

Patterson, James T.

1987   *The Dread Disease: Cancer and Modern American Culture*. Cambridge, Mass.: Harvard University Press.

Perin, Constance

1988   *Belonging in America: Reading between the Lines*. Madison: University of Wisconsin Press.

Peterson, Christopher, and Albert J. Stunkard

1989   "Personal Control and Health Promotion." *Social Science and Medicine* 28:819–28.

Pill, Roisin M., and Nigel C. H. Stott

1982   "Concepts of Illness Causation and Responsibility: Some Preliminary Data from a Sample of Working Class Mothers." *Social Science and Medicine* 16:43–52.

1985   "Choice or Chance: Further Evidence on Ideas of Illness and Responsibility for Health." *Social Science and Medicine* 20:981–91.

1987   "The Stereotype of 'Working-class Fatalism' and the Challenge for Primary Care Health Promotion." *Health Education Research* 2 (2):105–14.

Puska, Pekka, Kaj Koskela, Hilkka Pakarinen, Pirjo Puumalainen, Väinö Soininen, and Jaakko Tuomilehto

1976   "The North Karelia Project: A Programme for Community Control of Cardiovascular Diseases." *Scandinavian Journal of Social Medicine* 4:57–60.

Ragucci, Antoinette T.

1981   "Italian Americans." In *Ethnicity and Medical Care*. Alan Harwood, ed., pp. 211–63. Cambridge, Mass.: Harvard University Press.

Randall, Willard S., and Stephen D. Solomon

1977   *Building 6: The Tragedy at Bridesburg*. Boston: Little, Brown.

Rapp, Rayna

1988   "Chromosomes and Communication: The Discourse of Genetic Counseling." *Medical Anthropology Quarterly* 2:143–57.

Rebel, Hermann

1989 "Cultural Hegemony and Class Experience: A Critical Reading of Recent Ethnological-Historical Approaches." *American Ethnologist* 16:117–36 (part 1) and 350–65 (part 2).

Reed, Adolph, Jr.

1992 "The Underclass as Myth and Symbol: The Poverty of Discourse about Poverty." *Radical America* 24(1):20–40.

Reich, Robert B.

1987 *Tales of a New America.* New York: Times Books and Random House.

Richters, Arnis

1988 "Effects of Nitrogen Dioxide and Ozone on Blood-borne Cancer Cell Colonization of the Lungs." *Journal of Toxicology and Environmental Health* 25:383–90.

Rimer, B., W. Jones, C. Wilson, D. Bennett, and P. Engstrom

1983 "Planning a Cancer Control Program for Older Citizens." *Gerontologist* 23 (4):384–89.

Roberson, Nora

1987 "A Community-based Cancer Education Program." In *Public Education about Cancer: Recent Research and Current Programmes.* Patricia Hobbs, ed., pp. 33–40. UICC (International Union against Cancer) Technical Report Series, vol. 80. Toronto: Hans Huber Publishers.

Rosaldo, Michelle Z.

1984 "Toward an Anthropology of Self and Feeling." In *Culture Theory: Essays on Mind, Self, and Emotion.* Richard A. Shweder and Robert A. LeVine, eds., pp. 137–57. Cambridge: Cambridge University Press.

Rosaldo, Renato

1986 "From the Door of His Tent: The Fieldworker and the Inquisitor." In *Writing Culture: The Poetics and Politics of Ethnography.* James Clifford and George E. Marcus, eds., pp. 77–97. Berkeley: University of California Press.

Rosenman, Ray H., Richard J. Brand, C. David Jenkins, Meyer Friedman, Reuben Straus, and Moses Wurm

1975 "Coronary Heart Disease in the Western Collaborative Group Study: Final Follow-up Experience of 8 1/2 Years." *JAMA (Journal of the American Medical Association)* 233 (8):872–77.

Rosenstock, Irwin M.

1966 "Why People Use Health Services." *Milbank Memorial Fund Quarterly* 44 (3):94–124.

1974 "Historical Origins of the Health Belief Model." *Health Education Monographs* 2 (4):328–35.

Rubin, Lillian Breslow
1976   *Worlds of Pain: Life in the Working-class Family.* New York: Basic Books.

Rundall, Thomas G., and John R. C. Wheeler
1979   "The Effect of Income on Use of Preventive Care: An Evaluation of Alternative Explanations." *Journal of Health and Social Behavior* 20 (4):397–406.

Ryan, William
1976   *Blaming the Victim.* New York: Vintage Books, Random House.

Sacks, Karen Brodkin, and Dorothy Remy, eds.
1984   *My Troubles Are Going to Have Trouble with Me: Everyday Trials and Triumphs of Women Workers.* New Brunswick, N.J.: Rutgers University Press.

Said, Edward W.
1978   *Orientalism.* New York: Vintage Books, Random House.

Saillant, Francine
1990   "Discourse, Knowledge, and Experience of Cancer: A Life Story." *Culture, Medicine, and Psychiatry* 14 (1):81–104.

Saline, Carol, and the *Philadelphia Magazine* Staff
1981   "A Philadelphia-style Christmas." *Philadelphia Magazine* 72 (12):162–67.

Saline, Carol, Ron Javers, Polly Hurst, Mike Mallowe, Tom Moore, and Dorothy Cupich, eds.
1981   "Philadelphia Style." *Philadelphia Magazine* 72 (4):117–119.

Salzberger, Ruth Caro
1976   "Cancer: Assumptions and Reality Concerning Delay, Ignorance, and Fear." In *Social Anthropology and Medicine.* J. B. Loudon, ed., pp. 150–89. London: Academic Press.

Scheper-Hughes, Nancy, and Margaret M. Lock
1987   "The Mindful Body: A Prolegomenon to Future Work in Medical Anthropology." *Medical Anthropology Quarterly* 1:6–41.

Scotch, Norman
1963   "Sociocultural Factors in the Epidemiology of Zulu Hypertension." *American Journal of Public Health* 53 (8):1205–13.

Scott, James C.
1985   *Weapons of the Weak: Everyday Forms of Peasant Resistance.* New Haven: Yale University Press.

Shostak, Arthur B.
1980   *Blue-collar Stress.* Reading, Mass.: Addison-Wesley.

Singer, Merrill
1987   "Cure, Care, and Control: An Ectopic Encounter with Biomedical Obstetrics." In *Encounters with Biomedicine: Case Studies in Medical*

Anthropology. Hans A. Baer, ed., pp. 249–65. New York: Gordon and Breach.

Sontag, Susan
1977   *Illness as Metaphor*. New York: Random House.

Steward, David C., and Thomas J. Sullivan
1982   "Illness Behavior and the Sick Role in Chronic Disease: The Case of Multiple Sclerosis." *Social Science and Medicine* 16:1397–1404.

Taussig, Michael T.
1980   "Reification and the Consciousness of the Patient." *Social Science and Medicine* 14B:3–13.

Tepperman, Jean
1976   *Not Servants, Not Machines: Office Workers Speak Out!* Boston: Beacon Press.

Trostle, James A.
1988   "Medical Compliance as an Ideology." *Social Science and Medicine* 27 (12):1299–1308.

Urban Decision Systems, Inc.
1992   "Area Profile: 1990" and "Socio-economic Profile: 1990." Prepared for Philadelphia County and two 1990 census tracts. Los Angeles. Typescript.

U.S. Bureau of the Census
1972   *1970 Census of Population and Housing. Census Tracts, Philadelphia, Pa.–N.J. Standard Metropolitan Statistical Area*. Final Report PHC(1)-159. Washington, D.C.: Department of Commerce.
1983   *1980 Census of Population and Housing. Census Tracts, Philadelphia, Pa.–N.J. Standard Metropolitan Statistical Area*. PHC80–2-283. Washington, D.C.: Department of Commerce.

U.S. Centers for Disease Control
1991   *Health United States 1990*. National Center for Health Statistics, Public Health Service. DHHS Publication, no. 91–1232. Hyattsville, Md.: Department of Health and Human Services.

Valentine, Charles A.
1968   *Culture and Poverty: Critique and Counter-proposals*. Chicago: University of Chicago Press.

van Willigen, John
1986   *Applied Anthropology: An Introduction*. South Hadley, Mass.: Bergin and Garvey.

Wallerstein, Nina, and Edward Bernstein
1988   "Empowerment Education: Freire's Ideas Adapted to Health Education." *Health Education Quarterly* 15 (4):379–94.

Weiss, Leonard
1990   "Some Effects of Mechanical Trauma on the Development of Pri-

mary Cancers and Their Metastases." *Journal of Forensic Sciences* 35 (3):614–27.

West, Candace

1983 "'Ask Me No Questions . . . ': An Analysis of Queries and Replies in Physician-Patient Dialogues." In *The Social Organization of Doctor-Patient Communication.* Sue Fisher and Alexandra Dundas Todd, eds., pp. 75–106. Washington, D.C.: Center for Applied Linguistics.

White, Kerr L., ed.

1988 *The Task of Medicine: Dialogue at Wickenburg.* Menlo Park, Calif.: Henry J. Kaiser Family Foundation.

Willis, Paul E.

1977 *Learning to Labour: How Working Class Kids Get Working Class Jobs.* Westmead, Farnborough, England: Saxon House.

Wing, Steve

1988 "Social Inequalities in the Decline of Coronary Mortality." *American Journal of Public Health* 78:1415–16.

Workman, Stephen, Zili Amsel, Andrew Balshem, and Paul Engstrom

1988 "Cancer Control in a Defined Population: Results of the "Beat the Odds" Education Campaign." In *Advances in Cancer Control Research and the Emergence of the Oncology Product Line.* Paul F. Engstrom, Paul N. Anderson, and Lee E. Mortenson, eds., pp. 55–64. New York: Alan R. Liss.

Wulff, Robert M., and Shirley J. Fiske, eds.

1987 *Anthropological Praxis: Translating Knowledge into Action.* Boulder, Colo.: Westview Press.

Young, Allan

1980 "The Discourse on Stress and the Reproduction of Conventional Knowledge." *Social Science and Medicine* 14B:133–47.

Zola, Irving Kenneth

1972 "Medicine as an Institution of Social Control." *Sociological Review* 20 (4):487–504.

Academic anthropology, 133–36
Adherence (compliance): problems with, 6; professional authority and, 137
Air pollution. *See* Pollution
Alcohol use: in John's case, 102–3, 107, 109, 112; underreporting of, 112–13
American Anthropological Association meeting, 1–2, 10
American Public Health Association, 60
Anthropology: academic, 133–36; applied, 10–11, 128–36; authority in, 136–39, 143–44; reflexivity in, 125, 143–44
Applied anthropology: vs. academic, 133–36; conflicts in, 128–36
Asbestos, occupational exposure to, 24–25
Authority: vs. advocacy, 146; in anthropology, 136–39, 143–44; compliance and, 137; judgmental, 138, 147; of medical professionals, 113–14; morality of, 144; resistance to, 75–78, 86–88, 107–11, 117, 142

Belway Company, 38
"Big C, The," as metaphor, 79
Binzen, Peter, on life in river wards, 28

Cancer: attitudes toward, 45–54, 69–80; beliefs about causation of, 84–86; chemical plants' role in, 14, 17, 48–54; control of, 88–89; defiance against, 80–85; as devil's disease, 79; education on, 57–68; emotions evoked by, 72; environmental factors, 70–74, 103–5; fatalistic view of, 78–80; hesitancy to speak about, 79–80; impact on family, 116; incidence of, 17; lifestyle factors, 5–6, 31–32, 70–74, 103–5; misconceptions about, 64–66; mortality rates, 17, 19–20, 23–27; nonmedical resources against, 82–83; nutrition and, 59–60, 62; occupational risks for, 24–27; pollution and, 3, 8–9, 17–20, 24–27; 46–54; smoking and, 19–20, 75; as sneaky disease, 79; spread by surgery, 64, 66; as taboo, 80
Cancer clusters (hot spots), 17–20, 23–27
Caselli, Mary, 24–25
Chemical plants, 14, 17; explosion at, 48–54
Clifford, James, on ethnography, 129
Cobb, Jonathan, on power, 141
Communication deficits, between medical profession and community, 119–23

Compliance: problems with, 6; professional authority and, 137
Connors, Grandpa, 143
Consolidated Coke (industrial plant), 49
Control: of cancer, 88–89; by medical profession, 113–16; over health, pessimism on, 77–78; by working class, 85, 88–89
Cultural constructs, in patient-physician relationship, 119–23

"Dan," column by (*Guide* magazine), 32–39
Dayal, Hari, et al., study on cancer mortality rates, 19–20
Death, cancer seen as, 73
Deetz (industrial plant), 49
Defiance, against cancer, 80–85
Defiant ancestor, 80–85, 143
DiScala, Carla, 24
Disease, vs. illness, 119
Dorothy, assistance for, 40–41

Ecologic analysis, of cancer mortality rates, 19–20
Emotional issues: in cancer, 72, 116, 121, 123–24
Environmental factors: in cancer, 70–74, 103–5. *See also* Pollution
Explanatory Models (EM) concept, on cultural constructs of patient and physician, 119–23
Explosion, at chemical plant, 48–54

Family, cancer impact on, 116. *See also* Jennifer
Fatalism, 66–68, 73–74, 77–78, 87–88
Fishtown neighborhood, 29–30
Fox Chase Cancer Center: Department of Behavioral Science, 2–3; Project CAN-DO directed by, 55, 64, 126; research goals of, 4
Frykman, Jonas, on cultural hegemony, 141

General Chemical (industrial plant), 49–52
Gluckman, Max, on crossing separation of interests, 143–44

Gonzales, Juan, "The Cancer Zones" series by, 23–27
Government services, complaints about, 36–37
Gramsci, Antonio, on subordinate classes, 87
Guide, "by Dan" column in, 32–39

Health education: between community and scientific medicine, 126–27; judgment in, 145–46; moral dilemma in, 141; in Project CAN-DO, 57–68
Heart disease, questions on, in Project CAN-DO, 69–73
Hegemony, 87–88, 141
Herzfeld, Michael, 125, 142
Hospitals, cancer management in. *See under* John
Hughes, Dr., 111–24; as authority figure, 138; as victim, 142

Illness, vs. disease, 119
Industry, chemical, 14, 17, 48–54

Jackson, Michael, 125
Jennifer: on alcohol in John's medical record, 102–3, 122; autopsy and, 106–7, 109–10; conflict with Dr. Hughes, 111–18, 121–22; conflict with physicians, 96, 97; decisions on care, 114–15; dissatisfaction with hospitals, 93, 96, 97, 99, 100; emotional injury of, 122–24; Explanatory Models, 120–22; failure to see early symptoms, 94; in hero role, 119, 142; after John's death, 110–11; nervous state of, 98–99; resisting medical establishment dominance, 107–11, 117; satisfaction with Hospital F, 100, 101; on social class, 117–18; as Tannerstown resident, 92–93; as working-class representative, 138
John, 91–124; alcohol use by, 102–3, 107, 109, 112; autopsy on, 106–7, 109–10; cachexia in, 100; carcinoembryonic antigen levels of, 96; chemotherapy, 101; death, 105, 110; diagnosis, 98–100, 109; early life, 92–93; early symptoms, 94; environmental factors affecting, 104–5, 108–9; hallucinations, 99, 105; Hospital A (as emergency patient), 94;

Hospital B (weaker institution), 94–98, 107; Hospital C (teaching hospital), 95–98; Hospital D (small suburban), 96, 98–99, 107; Hospital E (with oncology program), 99–101; Hospital F (teaching hospital), 99–102, 107, 109, 110; illustrating communication deficits between community and clinic, 119–23; illustrating emotional issues, 123–24; illustrating working-class–medical establishment collision, 117–19; medical history, 102; medical record, 107–10; metastases diagnosed in, 101; onset of illness, 93–98; pain management for, 99, 100, 105; physician's view of, 111–24; seizure history, 102; smoking history, 95, 102, 104, 107, 108–10; social history, 102; social worker's notes on, 100–101; surgery, 98; terminal care, 102; wife of, *see* Jennifer; work history, 93; as working-class representative, 138; workplace accident, 103–4

Karp, Ivan, 125
Kensington neighborhood, 13, 28
Kleinman, Arthur, Explanatory Models concept, 119–23

Lifestyle factors, in cancer, 5–6, 24, 31–32, 70–74, 91, 103–5. *See also* Smoking
Lock, Margaret M., on medicalization, 67
Locus of health control, 153n3
Löfgren, Orvar, on cultural hegemony, 141

Mack, Kitty, 26
Mallowe, Mike, articles on river wards, 27–32
Marantz, Paul R., on blaming victim, 92
Martin, Emily, 9
Medicalization, 66–68
Medical profession: attitudes toward, 45–47; conflict with working class, 117–19; control by, 113–16; cultural constructs of, 119–23; dominance by, 107–11; lack of communication with, 119–

23; relationship with patient, 115; working-class representations of, 6–8
Melbourne company, 38
Mesothelioma, 24
Minkler, Meredith, on health education, 145–46
Morality, of authority, 144
Moral superiority, in anthropology, 135

National Cancer Institute, Project CAN-DO funding by, 55, 64
New England Journal of Medicine, 83
"New white ghetto," 27–32
Nutrition, cancer and, 59–60, 62

Occupational exposure: to asbestos, 24–25; to carcinogens, 24–27; to harmful substances, 14, 17, 48–54, 112

Pancreatic cancer, case study of. *See* John
Patient: cultural constructs of, 119–23; relationship with physician, 115
Peasants, control methods of, 87–88
Perin, Constance, on neighborly relations in suburbs, 33–34
Philadelphia: cancer hot spots in, 17–20, 23–27; cancer mortality rates in, 19; Kensington neighborhood, 13, 28. *See also* River wards; Tannerstown
Philadelphia Daily News, cancer zone series of, 23–27
Philadelphia Magazine, articles on river wards, 27–32
"Philadelphia Style" series, in *Philadelphia Magazine,* 29–31
Polk, Lewis, 25–26
Pollution: cancer and, 3, 8–9, 17–20, 24–27, 46–54; from chemical explosion, 48–54; community resistance to, 31, 38–39; government officials' denial of, 25–26; industry's denial of, 25; in river wards, 14, 26; in Tannerstown, 17
Praxis Award, Washington Area Practicing Anthropologists, 128
Preszinski, Della, 38
Professional authority. *See* Authority
Professionalism, vs. working class, 137–38
Project CAN-DO, 55–90, 126; anthropological aspects of, 69–90; as authority

figure, 138; baseline survey, 56, 60; community rejection of, 60–62; defiant ancestor invoked, 80–85; end of, 131–32; environmental factors in, 70–74; fatalistic responses in, 73–74, 78–80, 84–85; five-year plan, 56; focus groups, 69–70; health education, 57–68; heart disease questions, 69–73; interviews, 69–70; judgmental professional paradigm, 146; kickoff meeting, 63; lifestyle factors, 70–74; lottery, 61; mail survey, 56; misconceptions about cancer and, 64–66; nutrition survey in, 69; philosophy of, 64; public vs. individual discourses, 86–87; resistance demonstrated in, 75–78, 85–88; scope of, 55; special moments, 60–64; staffing, 55; typical educational event, 58–60

Reflexivity, in anthropology, 125, 143–44
Resistance: to authority, 75–78, 86–88, 107–11, 117, 142; of community to pollution, 31, 38–39; to medical establishment, 107–11, 117; in Project CAN-DO, 86, 87–88
Richters, Arnis, 8
River wards, 13: cancer rate opinions in, 54; crime in, 28; history, 13–14; *Philadelphia Magazine* articles on, 27–32; pollution in, 26; Project CAN-DO in, 55–90; urban decay in, 28–29, 31–32; variegated images of, 21–23. *See also* Tannerstown
Rosaldo, Michelle, on emotion, 121
Ryan, William, 5; on blaming victim, 5; on changing victim, 147

Said, Edward W., on beginning projects, 1
Scheper-Hughes, Nancy, on medicalization, 67
Scientific authority. *See* Authority
Scott, James C., on resistance in powerless groups, 87
Self-efficacy, 153n3
Sennett, Richard, on power, 141
Sister W., on socioeconomic conditions, 32
Smells, in Tannerstown, 49–50
Smoking: in "by Dan" column, 38; cancer and, 19–20, 75; in John's history, 95, 102, 104, 107, 108–10
Social class, 117–18; authority as dividing line for, 138; judging and, 138
Sontag, Susan, on cancer, 88
Surgery: cancer spread and, 64, 66; in John's case, 98

Tannerstown (pseudonym): air pollution in, 17; attitudes toward cancer in, 45–54; attitudes toward medical profession in, 7–8, 45–47; belonging in, 40–45; "by Dan" magazine column image of, 32–39; cancer beliefs of, 1–2; as "cancer hot spot," 17–20, 23–27; chemical plants in, 14, 17; community networks in, 42–44; Dayal study on, 19–20; demographics, 14–16; history, 13–14; images of, 20–39; as "new white ghetto," 27–32; physical borders, 41; pollution in, 18–20; Project CAN-DO in, *see* Project CAN-DO; religion in, 16–17; smells, 17, 49–50; social lives, 16–17; socioeconomic status, 16; as stable community, variegated images of, 21–23; view of outsiders, 45–54

Urban decay, 27–32

Valentine, Charles: on blaming victim, 5
Victimization, 76–77

Wallerstein, Nina, on health education, 146
Wanser (industrial plant), 49
Washington Area Practicing Anthropologists Praxis Award, 128
White ghetto, river wards as, 27–32
Whitetown USA (Binzen), 28
Willis, Paul E., on counter-school culture, 86
Working class: advocates for, 5; assumptions about, 5; complaints about government services by, 36–37; conflict with medical establishment, 117–19; fatalism of, 66, 67–68; generalizations about, 4–5; importance of social norms to, 32–33; intolerance of hypocrisy in, 37–38; lack of control by, 85, 88–89; as lower social class, 117–18; as model for

judged, 138; negative aspects of, 6; in "new white ghetto," 27–32; Philadelphians' perceptions of, 20–21; as problem, 5; vs. professionalism, 137–38; professional representations of, 4–6; representations of medical profession, 6–8; romance in, 34–35; roman-ticization of, 142; as social problem, 5; standards of house appearance in, 33–34; tradition of criticism, 7

Workplace exposure. *See* Occupational exposure

Yarbro, J. W., on carcinogenesis, 13